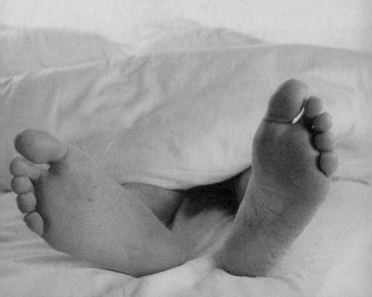

OVERCOMING
FATIGUE

In pursuit
of sleep
and energy

PAUL C. REISSER, M.D.

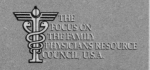

THE
FOCUS ON
THE FAMILY
PHYSICIANS RESOURCE
COUNCIL, U.S.A.

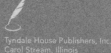

Tyndale House Publishers, Inc.
Carol Stream, Illinois

Visit Tyndale's exciting Web site at www.tyndale.com

TYNDALE is a registered trademark of Tyndale House Publishers, Inc.

Tyndale's quill logo is a trademark of Tyndale House Publishers, Inc.

Living Books is a registered trademark of Tyndale House Publishers, Inc.

Focus on the Family is a registered trademark of Focus on the Family, Colorado Springs, Colorado.

Overcoming Fatigue: In pursuit of sleep and energy

Designed by Luke Daab

Adapted from the *Complete Guide to Family Health, Nutrition, and Fitness* ISBN-10: 0-8423-6181-2; ISBN-13: 978-0-8423-6181-1. Copyright © 2006 by Tyndale House Publishers, Inc.

ISBN-13: 978-1-4143-1045-9
ISBN-10: 1-4143-1045-5

Printed in the United States of America

12 11 10 09 08 07 06
7   6   5   4   3   2   1

TABLE OF CONTENTS

FOREWORD BY
DR. JAMES DOBSON

August 15, 1990, began much like any other day for
me. I awoke early in the morning and headed to the
gym for a game of basketball with a group of friends
and colleagues—some of whom were as much as
twenty or thirty years younger than I! Because I frequently hit the court with these "youngsters," and
because I had reached middle age with the lanky build
that allowed me to still move easily, I assumed that I
was in the prime of physical health.

A sharp pain in my chest on that late summer morning told me otherwise. I excused myself from the game
and drove alone to the hospital (something I do *not* recommend to anyone who suspects he or she is experienc-
ing a serious medical problem!). Hoping and praying
that I was merely battling fatigue, I knew deep down
that there was something else terribly wrong. It didn't
take the doctors long to confirm that, sure enough, this
"healthy" basketball enthusiast had transformed, in the
blink of an eye, into a heart attack victim.

As I lay in the hospital in the days following that
ordeal, I realized that, early-morning basketball games
notwithstanding, my predicament was directly related to

my lifestyle choices and, in particular, the fatty foods I was allowing in my diet. I asked the Lord to give me another chance, resolving to use every resource at my disposal to safeguard my heart and my health through a combination of healthy diet and exercise. Despite some setbacks (I suffered a stroke in 1998 but recovered from it almost immediately), I have endeavored to keep that commitment, and, today, I am feeling better than ever.

Like so many Americans, prior to my heart attack, I was extremely busy—but not necessarily *active* in a way that would ensure optimal physical health. Indeed, statistics show that, despite our frantic pace of living and continued advances in the medical field, Americans suffer from an alarming number of health problems, many of which could be prevented or at least decreased by changing bad habits.

Research confirms just how serious the situation has become. The latest figures from the American Heart Association show that 13 million Americans have coronary heart disease; 5.4 million have suffered a stroke; and 65 million have been diagnosed with high blood pressure. Unfortunately, a large number of these cases are related, at least in part, to lifestyle choices. The AHA also reports that 48.5 million American adults (nearly 23 percent) are smokers. From 1995 to 1999, an average of 442,398 Americans died annually of smoking-related illnesses (32.2 percent of these deaths were cardiovascular related). The American Cancer

Society estimates that 180,000 of the cancer deaths in 2004 could be attributed to smoking. Further, one-third of cancer deaths in 2004 were related to nutrition, physical inactivity, being overweight or obese, and other lifestyle issues. In other words, many of them were *preventable*!

As I suggested earlier, perhaps the biggest factors in maintaining proper physical health are diet and exercise. Unfortunately, a recent study revealed that a full 25 percent of Americans reported participating in *no* physical activity during their leisure time. Perhaps that is why more than 65 percent of adults in the United States are overweight, including 30 percent who are clinically obese. Between 1971 and 2000, the average daily caloric intake for men grew by about 7 percent, which translates into seventeen pounds of additional body fat per year. Obesity dramatically affects life span as well. The life expectancy of a twenty-year-old white male who is clinically obese decreases by an estimated thirteen years, and for black males, an astonishing average of twenty years are lost due to obesity. One recent study revealed that the number of annual deaths attributable to obesity among adults in the United States is about 300,000. And perhaps most telling of all, airlines are telling us that they now have to carry additional fuel in order to transport more overweight customers.

This situation is sobering, but I am living proof that a dramatic change in eating habits, combined with a focused regimen of heart-strengthening exercise, can significantly improve one's overall health. I'll admit that the prospect of making such radical lifestyle changes can be daunting, but let me assure you that it is worth the investment. Choosing a healthy lifestyle *now*, while you still can, is infinitely preferable to being sidelined by a stroke, heart attack, cancer, or some other health crisis in the future.

This pocket guide and its parent book, the *Complete Guide to Family Health, Nutrition, and Fitness* are excellent resources designed to answer many of the questions that may arise as you endeavor to put yourself and your loved ones on the road to a healthier life. They can help you identify important medical tests; foster *emotional* and *spiritual* health in addition to physical fitness; discover answers to specific health-related questions for family members of all ages; and so much more. The information presented here is based on the most up-to-date medical research as well as the first-hand experiences of members of Focus on the Family's Physicians Resource Council. These experts will give you lots of practical advice on some critical disciplines.

Perhaps you consider yourself generally healthy and are simply looking for a plan to help you stay that way. Or maybe you or someone you love is suffering from a serious health problem related to poor lifestyle choices in the past. Either way, this book will provide you with the tools you need—as a complement to the advice of your personal physician, of course—to live smarter and healthier. Change is never easy, but it *is* possible, and I pray that God will bless you as you endeavor to be a good steward of the body He has given you.

James C. Dobson

James C. Dobson, Ph.D.

ACKNOWLEDGMENTS

The following members of the Focus on the Family Physicians Resource Council served as primary reviewers for all or parts of this manuscript, and their input, suggestions, and insights have been of critical importance:

BYRON CALHOUN, M.D., F.A.C.O.G., F.A.C.S.
Maternal-Fetal Medicine—Rockford, Illinois

DOUGLAS O. W. EATON, M.D.
Internal Medicine—Loma Linda, California

ELAINE ENG, M.D., F.A.P.A.
Psychiatry—Flushing, New York

J. THOMAS FITCH, M.D., F.A.A.P.
Pediatrics—San Antonio, Texas

DONALD GRABER, M.D.
Psychiatry—Elkhart, Indiana

W. DAVID HAGER, M.D., F.A.C.O.G.
Gynecology—Lexington, Kentucky

DANIEL R. HINTHORN, M.D., F.A.C.P.
Infectious Disease—Kansas City, Kansas

GERARD R. HOUGH, M.D., F.A.A.P.
Pediatrics—Brandon, Florida

GAYLEN M. KELTON, M.D., F.A.A.F.P.
Family Medicine—Indianapolis, Indiana

JOHN P. LIVONI, M.D.
Radiology—Little Rock, Arkansas

ROBERT W. MANN, M.D., F.A.A.P.
Pediatrics—Mansfield, Texas

MARILYN A. MAXWELL, M.D., F.A.A.P.
Internal Medicine/Pediatrics—St. Louis, Missouri

PAUL MEIER, M.D.
Psychiatry—Richardson, Texas

GARY MORSCH, M.D., F.A.A.F.P.
Family Medicine—Olathe, Kansas

MARY ANNE NELSON, M.D.
Family Medicine—Cedar Rapids, Iowa

GREGORY RUTECKI, M.D.
Internal Medicine—Columbus, Ohio

ROY C. STRINGFELLOW, M.D., F.A.C.O.G.
Gynecology—Colorado Springs, Colorado

MARGARET COTTLE, M.D.
Palliative Care—Vancouver, British Columbia

PETER NIEMAN, M.D., F.A.A.P.
Pediatrics—Calgary, Alberta

TYNDALE PUBLISHER

DOUGLAS R. KNOX

ACKNOWLEDGMENTS

EDITORIAL STAFF

PAUL C. REISSER, M.D.
Primary Author

DAVID DAVIS
Managing Editor/Contributing Author

LISA JACKSON
Tyndale Editor

FOCUS ON THE FAMILY

BRADLEY G. BECK, M.D.
Medical Issues Advisor/Research Editor/Contributing Author

VICKI DIHLE, PA-C
Medical Research Analyst/Contributing Author

BARBARA SIEBERT
Manager, Medical Outreach

LINDA BECK
Administrative Support

REGINALD FINGER, M.D.
Medical Issues Analyst

KARA ANGELBECK
Health and Wellness Coordinator

TOM NEVEN
Book Editor

WHY AM I SO TIRED ALL THE TIME?

Do any of the following situations sound familiar to you?

- Your hand "dive-bombs" the snooze button on your alarm several times every morning.
- You have trouble concentrating and find yourself nodding off during school or work.
- You often lie awake at night worrying about troubling issues or your schedule for the next day.
- You always seem to feel tired, no matter how long you sleep.

If so, you are not alone.

As many as one in four patients visiting a primary-care physician is likely to consider fatigue a significant problem, even when something else is the stated complaint.[1] Millions more who feel chronically tired still carry out their daily routines, whether out of habit, necessity, or self-discipline, even if they feel tired while doing it. For some, fatigue is so severe that they have difficulty fulfilling even their most basic responsibilities.

Medically speaking, fatigue is not a diagnosis but rather a symptom, one that may have numerous causes. When we say we're tired, we may in fact be referring to a number of different experiences: a transient feeling arising from a day of physical labor or a sleepless night, a symptom produced by a serious illness, drowsiness at some point in the day (or all day), or a generalized sense of feeling poorly that has lasted for months or years.

Feelings of fatigue originate from several sources: medical issues such as sleep disorders, personal choices such as overcommitment, and life circumstances such as raising small children. In some cases a simple adjustment can produce better sleep—turning on a fan to mute disrupting sounds, for example. In others, a medical examination or a close look at our lifestyle choices is in order.

In this book we'll explore many causes for fatigue, and we'll discuss ways to combat tiredness and renew energy. Before we do that, however, it's important to understand a bit about what happens during sleep. We'll take a brief look at how much sleep we need, what our bodies are doing when we sleep, and how we can get the most out of a night's slumber.

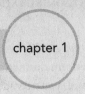

chapter 1

HOW MUCH SLEEP
DO I NEED?

The answer: Probably more than you are getting.

Sleep research has consistently shown that most adults actually *do* need the proverbial eight hours of sleep a night in order to perform at their best and avoid general tiredness, daytime drowsiness, and even fatigue-related illnesses. There are, of course, some who actually have a physiological need for as many as nine or ten hours and some who are fine on a routine of six or seven. The exact amount may be altered by genetics, sleep habits, and certain problems that can interfere with the quality of sleep.

The need for sleep varies as we age. Newborns often sleep twenty hours per day, while children may need anywhere from eight to thirteen hours (depending on age). Teenagers, who are notorious for gravitating toward a "late to bed and late to rise" schedule, also generally need nine hours. As we age, it's harder to fall asleep and stay asleep. Our sleep also tends to become less restful and more easily disrupted, and we spend less time in deeper phases of sleep.

How much sleep *you* need is best judged by how well you feel and perform during your waking hours. If you are sleep deprived, you may identify with one or more of these situations:

- You have come to hate whatever program is playing when your clock radio goes off.
- The first word out of your mouth upon arising is "Coffee . . ."
- You often feel sleepy and fatigued during the day.
- You have difficulty staying awake when you have to sit still, such as during a class or meeting or while driving.
- You struggle with irritability, poor concentration, or remembering facts.
- You find yourself relishing the chance to catch up on sleep on weekends or your day off.
- You fall asleep almost immediately when your head hits the pillow.

SLEEP DEBT AND SLEEP LATENCY

When a person fails to get the sleep that he or she needs for more than two or three days, whether due to an overextended lifestyle or a sleep disorder, that person begins to build what doctors call a sleep debt. Unfortunately, even with a steady flow of caffeine and a lot of activity, it's not really possible to adjust to sleeping fewer hours than are needed. As our sleep debt builds over several days, fatigue increases and mental and physical performance begin to suffer. The need for sleep will continue to grow until we sleep in on a weekend or a day off, become ill, or start napping during normal waking hours. In order to feel (and be) properly rested, the sleep debt will at some point need to be repaid. Sleep debt has been blamed for many major industrial and aviation accidents, and it is now implicated in overall poor health as well. The only way to repay a sleep debt is to get an hour or two more sleep than we typically need for several nights in a row—an assignment that can be surprisingly difficult. Once the debt has been dealt with, the brain reverts to seeking whatever amount of sleep it normally needs.

Fatigue and sleep debt also affect sleep latency, the actual amount of time it takes to fall asleep. If you're not fatigued or short on sleep, it can take twenty minutes or more to fall asleep. At the end of a long, demanding day, or with a buildup of sleep debt, sleep latency can shorten to a few minutes or less. If you experience a very short sleep latency night after night, this is usually an indication that the amount or quality of your sleep is inadequate. A short sleep latency should be noted as a warning sign, especially by anyone (such as a long-distance driver) whose life and safety depend upon staying awake.

If you have a restful vacation planned in the near future, try this experiment in order to help determine how much sleep you need on an ongoing basis: Once you are unpacked and settled in, go to bed each night when you feel tired and then sleep until you wake up spontaneously. Keep the room dark, set no alarms, and don't let other people awaken you. You may be paying back a sleep debt for several days, but after that you should start sleeping for about the length of time you actually need. If you don't have a vacation planned soon or will be following a busy itinerary on your next trip, you can try a similar experiment at home. Try to go to bed about fifteen minutes earlier each night (fifteen minutes the first night, thirty minutes the second night, and so on) until you discover the amount of sleep that leaves you feeling completely restored the next day.

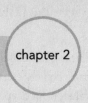

chapter 2

WHAT HAPPENS
WHEN I SLEEP?

The brain is undergoing all kinds of activity while asleep, cycling repeatedly through phases of sleep known as stages 1, 2, 3, 4, and REM (rapid eye movement). The first four stages, together called non-REM sleep, make up about 75 percent of our sleep time. The quality of our sleep—the correct amount, proportion, and patterns of REM and non-REM sleep—is as important as the total amount of sleep.

The first and lighter phases of non-REM sleep are stages 1 and 2. When we struggle to stay awake and keep nodding off, we may drift in and out of stage 1 sleep, from which it is easiest to awaken. During this stage, our eyes often move and muscles twitch, and we may even remember some images ("I got so drowsy that I was starting to dream . . . "), but this in fact is not the stage in which we do our dreaming. We spend about 50 percent of our total sleep time in stage 2, when eye movements and brain waves slow down. From there we progress to stages 3 and 4, known as deep sleep, which is the most restorative. Blood pressure, pulse, and breathing rates all decrease, and eye movements and muscle activity essentially stop. It is more difficult to awaken from deep sleep, and when it is interrupted, we may feel groggy or even disoriented for several minutes. Bed-wetting, sleepwalking, and night terrors in children occur during stages 3 and 4.

Rapid eye movement sleep—so named because our eyes move actively under the eyelids during this phase—is the stage during which we dream. Breathing becomes more rapid and less regular, and arms and legs become temporarily paralyzed as the brain electrically disconnects from the spinal cord and stops sending messages to the muscles. This is an important safeguard because when it fails, people literally act out their dreams, often with disastrous results.

When we first fall asleep, we generally pass through stages 1 through 4 in sequence, then return to the lighter phases of sleep, from which we enter the first REM phase about sixty to ninety minutes after dozing off. Brain waves slow down more and more as we pass from stage 1 through stage 4. But during REM sleep, brain-wave activity is very similar to what occurs when we're awake. We continue cycling through the non-REM stages during the night, interrupted by periods of REM, each complete cycle lasting around 90 to 110 minutes. During the first of these, the deeper stages of sleep last longer with a relatively short period (fifteen to twenty minutes) of REM sleep.

As we continue through the night, REM becomes more predominant and deep sleep less so, such that sleep cycles closer to morning consist almost entirely of stages 1 and 2 and REM sleep. This is an important observation, because those of us who are getting only five or six hours of sleep per night may be unintentionally eliminating a significant amount of our much-needed REM sleep.

Many factors and a number of sleep disorders can disrupt the pattern of a person's sleep stages, so that he or she can actually sleep for what seems to be a reasonable amount of time but still feel exhausted and drowsy the next day. Imagine (or remember) being awakened every thirty minutes during the night by a barking dog or a crying child. Even if you fell asleep fairly quickly after each interruption, you would need to reenter sleep through stage 1, then cycle into the other stages. Since it usually takes at least thirty to forty minutes to enter the deeper, restorative phases of sleep and REM, you would have difficulty reaching them. In the morning you would probably feel pretty miserable, even if you managed to cobble together seven or eight hours of sleep, because the quality of your sleep would have been disrupted.

chapter 3

HOW CAN I GET A GOOD NIGHT'S SLEEP?

The following recommendations are the ABC's of a good night's rest and the first steps to review when insomnia becomes an issue:

1. Establish consistent sleep and wake-up times that provide enough sleep *every* day—and thus don't change radically on weekends or days off.

2. Develop a "winding down" routine that serves as a cue for your mind and body to get ready for sleep. This might include a warm bath, some diverting or inspirational reading, or pleasant music (but *not* the evening news, which is routinely jammed with the most lurid, disturbing, and unpleasant events of the day). An uplifting psalm or other Scripture passage containing some spiritual good news will provide better raw material for your sleeping brain to process.

3. Exercising regularly is helpful for a good night's sleep, but try to avoid vigorous activity within three hours of bedtime. This raises body temperature and tends to stimulate the brain rather than sedate it—

which is why morning is a better time for your workout. Your body cools down (a condition more favorable to sleep) about five to six hours after exercise, so a late-afternoon or even early evening workout can be conducive to sleep.

4. If at all possible, avoid personal turbulence prior to bedtime. If you have an important issue to discuss with someone (especially your spouse), don't start the conversation at bedtime. Fatigue at the end of the day (and the irritability, frustration, and short tempers that accompany it) will not only lead to a full-blown argument but also generate enough agitation to interfere with sleep. Schedule the conversation for a time and place when you are both rested and calm.

5. Avoid going to bed hungry or shortly after a large meal. A feast before bedtime may provoke heartburn or bloating, and the liquids that typically accompany it may fill up the bladder during the night. Some people, however, find that a light snack at bedtime helps them fall asleep more easily.

6. Make your sleeping area as quiet, dark, and comfortable as possible, avoiding extremes in temperature. Most sleep experts recommend sleeping in a cooler room rather than a warm one, because a hot environment tends to cause lighter sleep and more awakenings during the night.

7. Avoid caffeine (not only in coffee, but also in tea, soft drinks, and even chocolate), nicotine (from

smoking or patches/gum), or alcohol late in the day. Caffeine and nicotine are stimulants that tend to keep you awake, and alcohol, while initially sedating, interferes with sleep patterns.

8. Don't use your bed for anything other than sexual relations or sleep. Your bed isn't meant to be your office, your TV viewing area, or the place in which you unravel the mysteries of your life. Attempting to deal with work tasks and other issues in your bed can definitely interfere with relaxing and falling asleep.

9. If you can't sleep after thirty or forty minutes, don't continue to lie awake in bed. Get up and do some sort of relaxing activity, such as reading (something rather boring might be helpful) or listening to calming music, until you get sleepy. Try not to solve the world's problems, or your own, in the middle of the night. If some issue has you pacing the floor when everyone else is asleep, write a short list of specific "action items" that will help you deal with it the next day, and then go to bed. When you are tempted to revisit the problem instead of sleeping, remember that you now have a to-do list . . . for tomorrow . . . in another room. Now it's time to rest. If you truly cannot stop the flow of thoughts racing through your head during the night, you may need some help from your physician.

10. If you have trouble falling asleep night after night, avoid daytime napping, which can delay the onset of

sleep later. However, napping can be a useful short-term strategy when you know you won't be getting much sleep that night or when you have an accumulating sleep debt.

MAKING THE MOST OF A NAP

You may be surprised to learn that a brief "power nap" may be as refreshing as a two-hour snoozefest. Sleep research suggests that a short nap can improve performance and alertness, sharpen memory, and delay the need for sleep later in the day. An effective short nap should typically last no longer than twenty minutes. If you sleep longer, you are likely to enter the deeper phases of sleep from which it is much more difficult to awaken and stay alert.

Napping is usually easier during the period of normal sleepiness that occurs from about two to five in the afternoon. If you have a significant sleep debt, then napping as long as one-and-a-half to two hours will allow you to pass through a complete REM cycle, providing more rest and making it easier to wake up.

chapter 4

WHAT FACTORS CAN DISRUPT SLEEP?

Our circumstances and habits can cheat us of restorative sleep. Before we look at these sleep disrupters, however, we need to introduce an important factor that impacts our patterns of sleeping and waking: our circadian rhythm. Derived from Latin words meaning "around the day," this term refers to changes in the physiology of our body that occur in roughly twenty-four-hour cycles. The internal clock that drives the circadian rhythm is a pair of tiny structures called the suprachiasmatic nuclei, or SCN, that direct some two hundred circadian fluctuations, including variations in our blood pressure, body temperature, and hormone levels. Their location in the brain—just above the area at which the optic nerves cross—is strategic in that they receive input from the eyes as to the presence of light and darkness.

During the day the SCN signal a structure called the pineal gland to reduce the production of melatonin, a hormone that increases drowsiness. Rising levels of melatonin after dark help induce sleepiness. For most people, circadian-driven sleep-wake patterns linked to darkness and light cause a marked increase in the desire to sleep between midnight and 6 A.M. (no great surprise) and bring about another drowsy period during the midafternoon. The tradition of an afternoon nap or siesta in some cultures undoubtedly arises from a combination of this normal fluctuation in sleepiness and the burden of laboring or conducting business during the heat of the day.

ENVIRONMENTAL FACTORS

Environmental factors are notorious for disturbing sleep. A barking dog, crying baby, noisy neighbor, thunderstorm, police siren, or other unpredictable racket can cause one or more awakenings.

One type of noise that few people become accustomed to is the snoring of a bedmate, especially if it comes in fits and starts throughout the night. (Snoring may be caused by sleep apnea, which is discussed in more detail in chapter 6.) Someone whose sleep is particularly sensitive to noise might have to take measures to block unwanted sounds (such as using earplugs) or to mask them using a device that generates neutral sound (white noise) or simulates a pleasant sonic environment, such as a mountain stream or breeze in a forest.

Too much light in a room can interfere with sleep. A room that is too hot, too cold, or too stuffy will also keep slumber at bay. High altitude can interfere with the quality and quantity of sleep for a few nights until a person becomes accustomed to it. Many people who have adapted to a particular set of surroundings (especially their own mattress) might also have considerable difficulty falling asleep or staying asleep in a hotel or guest room.

POPULAR HABITS

A number of popular habits can disrupt sleep. Caffeine is well-known for its mild stimulant effects, but for some a cup of coffee or a caffeinated soft drink can promote wakefulness for up to twelve hours. Tobacco use can interfere with sleep because of nicotine's stimulant effects. Alcohol has a temporary sedating effect, depending upon the amount consumed, but it can lead to frequent waking later in the night. A large meal eaten shortly before retiring can lead to reflux—a backflow of stomach acid into the esophagus—and heartburn during the night.

AGING

Aging is frequently associated with disturbed sleep: More than 50 percent of people over age sixty-five report some type of sleep problem. Seniors are more likely to have difficulty falling asleep, spend less time in the deeper stages of sleep, experience early morning awakening, and accrue less total time asleep. Contrary to a commonly held notion, the elderly do not need less sleep. Instead, they more frequently experience decreased sleep efficiency and are vulnerable to more factors that can impair sleep. These include:

- Poor sleep habits, including irregular sleep-wake times and daytime napping, that interfere with falling asleep at night.
- Acute and chronic illnesses, and the medications that treat them.
- Significant social changes, usually involving profound personal losses, such as leaving a familiar home and community, the death of a loved one, separation from loved ones and friends, a move to a long-term care facility, and so on.
- Emotional upheavals, including anxiety and depression, as well as changes in overall mental function. Dementia (deteriorating cognitive abilities stemming from Alzheimer's disease, stroke, and other illnesses) often is accompanied by agitation, disorientation, and disruptive behaviors at night that wreak havoc on sleep, not only for the individual but also for his or her live-in caregivers.

SHIFT WORK

Studies of night-shift workers almost always reveal significant disruptions of circadian rhythms, including circadian dysynchrony, in which the various cycles of blood pressure, temperature, alertness, and hormone secretion are out of sync not only with the clock but with each other as well.

Shift workers can have particular trouble if they don't avoid sunlight, because the pattern of outside light and darkness is a powerful cue to the internal clock. As we just mentioned, normal circadian physiology causes most people to gravitate to a pattern of wakefulness during the day and sleep at night—the opposite of the night-shift work schedule. When they get a day or two off, many who have worked several consecutive night shifts may try to stay awake during the day in order to spend time with family and friends. Then it's back to the night shift.

Not surprisingly, attempting to adjust the circadian rhythm so quickly usually results in drowsiness at work and insomnia at home. As many as 10 to 20 percent of night-shift workers report falling asleep on the job, especially toward the end of the shift. Overall they tend to get five to seven fewer hours of sleep each week compared to their counterparts on day or evening shifts. As a result, night-shift workers are at an increased risk not only for health problems (including heart disease, digestive disorders, and disturbances), but also for more frequent and serious accidents. The Three Mile Island and Chernobyl nuclear-power-plant accidents, the *Exxon Valdez* oil spill, and the Bhopal, India, chemical gas leak that killed 3,800 people all occurred during the night shift and have been attributed, at least in part, to errors made by fatigued workers.

Help for the night crew

If you are a shift worker who must sleep during the day, you have two major challenges: limiting the day-light cues that tell your circadian clock to stay awake and minimizing the interruptions to your sleep when others are up and about. These mean:

- If you're going to sleep in the morning after a night shift, wear dark glasses on the way home and keep your exposure to the morning daylight to a minimum.
- Keep your bedroom dark, quiet, and at a comfortable temperature.
- Turn the phone off in your bedroom.
- Ask family members to do their best to keep noise levels down. Wear earplugs if necessary.

Your other major concern is staying awake and safe on the job. To the degree that your job, workplace, and employer permit, the following can help you:

- Keep your work area as well lit as possible.
- Talk with coworkers to help keep you alert.
- Move around briefly and stretch as often as possible, especially if you start to feel drowsy.
- If your routine is to sleep soon after your shift is over, and if you use coffee or other caffeinated beverages, try to avoid drinking them late in the shift. (A mug of coffee at 6 A.M. may make it difficult to fall asleep at home a couple of hours later.)
- If possible, walk briskly or do some other light exercise during your breaks.
- If your job involves tasks that are particularly boring, try to do them when you are most alert (which is usually early in the shift).

Don't forget about safety on the way home. If you carpool, let the person who feels (and acts) the most alert do the driving, and help to keep that person engaged in conversation. If you have a lengthy solo drive and repeatedly fight drowsiness behind the wheel, consider a short nap before leaving work, look into carpooling, or even consider public transportation.

One other important recommendation for shift workers that can be particularly tough to follow is going to bed at the same time every day—even on days off or weekends, when you want to get other things done during the day. This can help prevent seesawing circadian rhythm disruptions.

JET LAG

Jet lag is a common sleep disruption brought about by flying long distances. After a flight across several time zones, a person's circadian rhythm suddenly becomes out of sync with the local time. Depending on the number of time zones changed, the length of travel, and the level of sleep deprivation associated with the trip, jet lag can significantly affect a person's mental performance, sleep-wake cycle, and general well-being for several days after arrival. Symptoms of jet lag include irritability, fatigue, daytime drowsiness, poor concentration, intestinal disturbances (including diar-rhea), and nighttime awakening. Most people find that jet lag is more troublesome when traveling eastward than westward. Generally it takes about one day to adjust for each time zone traveled east or west. (When a person travels north or south along a time zone, there is generally no disruption to the circadian rhythm, though the traveler may still be tired from making the trip.)

Beating and treating jet lag

Seasoned travelers have learned several techniques that speed the alignment of their circadian rhythm with the local time zone. These include:

- If you have a few days to prepare for a west-to-east cross-country flight, try to synchronize your inner clock with your destination's time zone over three or more successive nights. If your normal bedtime is midnight, go to bed at 11 P.M. one night, 10 P.M. the next, and then 9 P.M. for a night or two. If you can get up earlier as well, even better. When the time comes to fly to the east coast, you'll be less likely to lie awake at midnight (9 P.M. Pacific time) and then wonder what hit you when the alarm goes off at 7 A.M. (4 A.M. Pacific).

- Transatlantic west-to-east flights cover even more time zones, so resynchronizing can be challenging. If you can travel on an overnight flight and sleep for a few hours on the plane, the transition will be much easier. (This may require a little help from your doctor in the form of a short-acting sleeping medication, assuming that its use is appropriate for your current health status.) An alternative is to arrange your flight(s) so that you arrive in the evening, and then go to bed at 10 or 11 P.M. If you arrive earlier and need to nap, avoid sleeping more than two hours.

- As soon as you depart, set your watch for the time zone of your destination.
- Avoid common sleep disrupters for a few hours prior to bedtime at your destination. These include alcohol, caffeine, nicotine, or intense exercise.
- Once you have arrived, get outside during the day as much as possible in order to cue your brain to the current timing of day and night.
- Melatonin supplementation has been widely promoted as a treatment for jet lag and appears to be helpful at least for some long-distance travelers. It is typically taken for a few days after arrival, in doses of 1 to 3 mg about a half hour before going to bed. Melatonin's safety during pregnancy or while nursing has not been established, and it is not recommended for long-term use.

chapter 5

WHAT SHOULD
I DO WHEN I CAN'T
FALL ASLEEP?

Few experiences in life are as frustrating as lying awake
at night unable to sleep, periodically glancing at a bedroom clock that delivers nothing but bad news. *It's
3:15? I'm supposed to be up in less than four hours! This is
going to be one rotten day!* Insomnia is generally defined
as the awareness of having trouble getting to sleep or
staying asleep, or the perception of not sleeping well
and not waking up refreshed.

Insomnia is often categorized by its duration: transient, short-term, or chronic. *Transient* insomnia lasts a
few nights and is generally caused by stress, jet lag,
changes in sleep timing, or an alteration of the sleep
environment. Many people, especially as they get older,
become so accustomed to the feel of their own bed that
an overnight stay anywhere else—whether in a hotel,
guest room, campground, or hospital—becomes an
ordeal until they become acclimated to the new surroundings. *Short-term* insomnia is poor sleep lasting two
to three weeks, often caused by stress, medical issues, or

psychological problems. Addressing the cause will usually bring sleep back to normal. *Chronic* insomnia involves difficulty falling or staying asleep that continues for a month or longer—sometimes *much* longer. This is usually related to an underlying medical, behavioral, or psychological problem such as depression.

It is important to note that insomnia is a symptom, like headache or fatigue, that can have many different characteristics, causes, and possible treatments. If the cause is readily identifiable and self-limited, no specific evaluation or treatment may be necessary. But if insomnia is a recurrent or chronic event, it should not—and usually cannot—be ignored. Very often the solution may be a simple one: taming a caffeine habit, for example, or acquiring a pair of earplugs to reduce the impact of a spouse's snoring, which itself may need to be evaluated. If you or a loved one is struggling with insomnia, *a review of sleep habits should be the first order of business*. (See chapter 3, beginning on page 9.)

SLEEP MEDICATIONS

A common response among people who are dealing with insomnia is to try some form of self-medication. One of the most common methods (and definitely a bad one) is a nightcap, an alcoholic beverage at bedtime. Needless to say, alcohol is definitely not a good choice for a sleep aid. While it may induce a little drowsiness, alcohol actually keeps some people awake. It suppresses REM sleep until it is metabolized, delaying this phase until later at night. It can also cause more frequent waking (including an additional trip or two to the bathroom), thus reducing the overall quality of sleep.

The most common nonprescription medication is the antihistamine diphenhydramine, sold as Benadryl (and other brands) and commonly found in "PM" forms of cold and pain relievers. A dose of 25 to 50 mg of diphenhydramine commonly brings on drowsiness, which makes it a poor choice for treating allergies during the day. (Some people, however, do not become sleepy on this medication.) Another sedating antihistamine is doxylamine, which is usually found in nonprescription cold remedies such as NyQuil. Either of these antihistamines can help induce sleep, and they're particularly useful if a person has both allergic symptoms and insomnia. However, they can also have an effect lasting beyond the sleep period and may cause daytime drowsiness the next day. They may also interfere with sleep patterns, resulting in a poorer quality of sleep. People with asthma or chronic lung disease should avoid these medications because they can thicken respiratory secretions, and men with symptoms arising from an enlarged prostate may have difficulty passing urine when taking one.

Many people who struggle with insomnia have tried taking melatonin, which can be purchased at any supermarket or pharmacy without a prescription. As we mentioned earlier, melatonin is a hormone that is known to induce drowsiness. Produced by the pineal gland within the brain, it normally increases during the night and falls to very low, almost undetectable levels during the day. Taken about thirty minutes before bedtime in doses from 1 to 3 mg (although the optimal dose is unknown), melatonin induces drowsiness in many individuals. It is also used by travelers as a treatment for jet lag, and it may help synchronize a person's circadian rhythm to the local time zone. But very few studies have examined melatonin's side effects, its interactions with other drugs, or the consequences of taking it on a long-term basis. Also, because there is very little regulation of the manufacture of herbal and food supplements, the amount and quality of melatonin may vary among the many formulations currently on the market.

Valerian, an extract of the root of the valerian plant, has a mildly relaxing effect and has been utilized widely in Europe as a treatment for insomnia. Its effects may not be noticeable for several days or even a few weeks, and thus it would not likely prove useful for transient or short-term insomnia. Because valerian may boost the effects of other sedating medications or alcohol, you should not take it with these drugs. Many preparations are available, and as with melatonin, quality and exact quantity may vary among them. A typical dose is 400 to 500 mg taken one or two hours before bedtime. (One major U.S. pharmaceutical company has entered this herbal arena with a valerian preparation called Alluna.)

Several types of prescription medications have been used to promote and maintain sleep. One class of drugs, the barbiturates (such as Nembutal, or pentobarbital), was widely used a few decades ago but is prescribed far less frequently today. Barbiturates adversely affect the quality of sleep, have significant side effects, tend to be addictive (both psychologically and physically), and can be extremely dangerous when taken in an overdose.

A class of drugs called benzodiazepines is well known for its members that reduce anxiety: diazepam (Valium), alprazolam (Xanax), lorazepam (Ativan), and clonazepam (Klonopin). All of these are sedating to some degree, and many people who take them for anxiety also use a bedtime dose to help with sleep. Other benzodiazepines that produce overt drowsiness have been widely prescribed as sleeping medications. The most common of these are triazolam (Halcion), temazepam (Restoril), and flurazepam (Dalmane). Estazolam (ProSom) and quazepam (Doral) are used less often. These medications vary dramatically in the duration of their activity:

- Triazolam takes effect relatively quickly and then wears off in about four hours, making it an ideal drug for inducing sleep on an overnight cross-country or transoceanic flight.

Typical doses are 0.125 or 0.25 mg. Taking more than 0.25 mg is not recommended: When the drug was first introduced, a 0.5 mg dose was available, but its use was found to be associated with amnesia and erratic behavior.

- The effects of temazepam extend over about eight hours, which makes it more useful for people who have trouble both falling and staying asleep.

- Flurazepam stays in the bloodstream for so long that a person taking it for the first time may be groggy for much of the next day. Even if that doesn't occur, flurazepam tends to accumulate in the body if taken over several successive nights, which can lead to persistent daytime sedation. The elderly are particularly vulnerable to this consequence.

While no sleeping medication is recommended for long-term use, the sedating benzodiazepines are particularly ill suited for this role because they tend to interfere with sleep patterns, thus affecting the overall quality of sleep. Ongoing use can also lead to rebound insomnia, an unpleasant worsening of sleeplessness when the drug is discontinued. These medications should never be taken with alcohol because the combination can cause excessive sedation (including suppression of respiration), and they can be hazardous when taken in an overdose.

These problems with benzodiazepines have fueled interest in a new class of sleeping medications that are much safer and do not seem to affect sleep patterns. The three forms currently available, zolpidem (Ambien), zaleplon (Sonata), and eszopiclone (Lunesta), are effective for most people and do not appear to be physically addictive. Like any sleeping medication, however, ongoing use can lead to psychological dependence: *I've run out of my pills. . . . I won't be able to sleep tonight!* Also, until they become available in generic forms, they will be much more expensive than the benzodiazepines.

Sleep experts routinely counsel against using any sleeping medication regularly for more than a few weeks, if that long. There are a number of reasons for this. Long-term use may result in psychological and even physical dependence, disruption of sleep patterns (though not with zolpidem, zaleplon, and eszopiclone), daytime sedation (with longer-acting drugs), and adverse interactions with other medications. More importantly, treating chronic insomnia with sleeping medications is not appropriate if the reason for the problem has not been explored. If someone has wakeful nights because of depression, for example, a prescription for sleeping pills will treat only one symptom and not the underlying problem.

chapter 6

DO I HAVE A SLEEP DISORDER?

Sleep specialists frequently distinguish between insomnia, the general feeling of not getting enough (or good quality) sleep, and sleep disorders, which are specific abnormalities in the physiology of sleep that can affect its duration and quality. An estimated 40 million Americans suffer from one of more than eighty identified sleep disorders. These are responsible for many cases of chronic insomnia, but few of the millions of people who have transient or short-term insomnia have an identifiable or diagnosable sleep disorder.

DIAGNOSING SLEEP DISORDERS

If a significant sleep problem lasts more than a week, you should see a health-care provider for an evaluation. (For more on how to prepare for an examination see chapter 8, "When Should I Consult a Doctor?") In some situations your doctor might refer you to a physician with special training in managing sleep problems, if one is available in your area.

One of the most widely used (but by no means simplest) steps in diagnosing a sleep disorder is a sleep study (called polysomnography). This usually involves an overnight stay in a sleep laboratory, which may be set up in a specialist's office or in a center utilized by many physicians. During such a study, a person sleeps in a private room that is monitored by closed-circuit television and microphones. Sensors attached to the head and face using nonallergic tape record brain waves and eye movements. Other skin sensors detect muscle activity. Elastic bands around the chest and abdomen track respirations. A special clip on one finger measures oxygen levels and heart rate.

It takes about an hour to make all these preparations, none of which are painful. While falling asleep under such unfamiliar circumstances would seem to be challenging, the vast majority of people who need a sleep study don't usually lie awake all night in the lab.

Some organizations offer sleep studies in the home, which sound appealing in many respects but may or may not provide the quantity and quality of information that can be obtained in a fully equipped lab. Before having a home study done, a person should confirm that both the provider and the physician interpreting the study are properly credentialed. Because a sleep study can be expensive (five hundred to one thousand dollars or more), it is also important to check with one's medical insurance provider before having it done, because many plans have restrictions or may require prior authorization. Some common sleep disorders are sleep apnea, narcolepsy, parasomnias, and delayed sleep phase syndrome.

SLEEP APNEA

It is estimated that as many as 18 million Americans have sleep apnea, which is characterized by interruptions of breathing lasting ten seconds or longer (in some cases, up to two minutes). By far the most common form is called obstructive sleep apnea (OSA), which occurs when soft tissues at the back of the nose, mouth, and throat relax during sleep, gradually obstructing the passage of air flowing into the upper airway. People with this disorder often snore loudly, and as their airways become more obstructed during sleep, the snoring becomes even more pronounced, until breathing stops. The short lapse in breathing causes the level of oxygen in the blood to drop precipitously. This provokes an arousal from sleep, during which the person gasps, coughs, chokes, or snorts as the obstruction clears and breathing resumes. It is possible for breathing to slow down without stopping, which is called hypopnea. The severity of sleep apnea is determined by the number of episodes of apnea or hypopnea per hour (five to fifteen is mild, sixteen to thirty is moderate, and more than thirty episodes per hour is severe), as well as by the level to which blood oxygen levels drop during the episodes.

A person may slow or stop breathing hundreds of

times during the night without awakening and will rarely if ever remember any of these episodes (although he or she may drive a spouse seeking some peace and quiet into another room). Remembered or not, such episodes repeatedly disrupt the normal transitions between sleep stages and the amount of time spent in each sleep phase, so that a person with OSA is usually sleep deprived even if logging eight or more hours in bed. The obvious consequence is fatigue and drowsiness during the day, especially when sitting still. People with OSA are at increased risk for having an accident at work or while driving, and those with severe cases may actually fall asleep while eating or talking.

Other medical problems linked to sleep apnea are equally important. As many as 50 percent of people with this disorder have high blood pressure (hypertension). Oxygen levels sag whenever breathing stops, which can provoke potentially dangerous irregular heart rhythms, as well as an increased risk for heart attack in people with coronary artery disease. Stroke is also linked to sleep apnea.

You might have sleep apnea if . . .
Several factors put people at risk for having sleep apnea, including:
- **Age.** Most people with this condition are over thirty (although children can have this problem as well).
- **Gender.** Men are three times more likely to have this problem than women.

- **Ethnicity.** Sleep apnea is more common among African-Americans, Hispanics, and Pacific Islanders.
- **Obesity.** Most people with this problem are overweight.
- **Neck size.** The presence of extra tissue in obese people can obstruct airflow. The risk for sleep apnea is higher for men whose neck circumference is greater than seventeen inches (for women, greater than sixteen inches).
- **Excessive soft tissue in the mouth and throat.** Enlarged tonsils and adenoids (especially in children), a prominent uvula (the "punching bag" that hangs from the back of the palate), or a large tongue increases the risk.
- **Sleep position.** Sleeping on one's back and using multiple pillows aggravate the collapse of soft tissues that obstruct airflow.
- **Use of alcohol or other sedatives before bedtime.**
- **Smoking.**

The above risk factors do not guarantee that sleep apnea is present, but the following symptoms should definitely raise one's suspicions:

- **Loud snoring during the night and drowsiness during the day.** Not everyone who snores has sleep apnea, nor does everyone who is sleepy during the day. But when these two symptoms occur together, sleep apnea is a very strong possibility.
- **Episodes in which breathing stops for ten seconds or more,** whether a few or many times per hour, especially if they end with gasping or other distressing sounds. Obviously, these must be heard by someone else.

Several other symptoms are common with sleep apnea, but these can have other causes:

- Rarely, if ever, feeling refreshed after sleeping
- Poor concentration, irritability, and fatigue during the day
- Morning headaches
- Tossing and turning during the night

In children, symptoms may be less obvious. Snoring may be present but daytime drowsiness may not. Parents may also notice restless sleep, frequent waking, and poor school performance.

Treatments for sleep apnea

A person who thinks he or she may have sleep apnea should undergo a thorough medical evaluation, not only to assess the primary complaints but also because other health problems (such as high blood pressure, heart disease, and obesity) will usually need to be addressed as well. A sleep study can provide both the diagnosis and an opportunity to try, if appropriate, a widely used treatment option called continuous positive airway pressure, or CPAP, which can be very helpful for those with moderate to severe sleep apnea. CPAP involves wearing a face mask, with straps extending around the head, that is connected to a machine that increases air pressure in the mouth and throat. This helps keep air passages open and thus reduces or prevents the episodes of obstruction. While using such a contraption during the night may sound unpleasant, most people with sleep apnea do become accustomed to it. More importantly, they nearly always notice an immediate and dramatic improvement the next day: a sense of feeling refreshed, alert, and energetic, and often relieved of morning headaches as well.

Other approaches to treating sleep apnea include:

- **Losing excess weight.** While easier said than done, this can make a definite difference in both sleep and a number of other health problems.
- **Sleeping on one's side.** One low-tech approach involves attaching a tennis ball to the back of a person's pajama top, either by creating a pocket for it or (for those lacking sewing skills) using duct tape. This simple but effective annoyance prevents one from sleeping on his or her back and therefore keeps the airways unobstructed.
- **Avoiding alcohol and other sedatives, especially before bedtime.**
- **Relieving chronic nasal congestion** with decongestants, cortisone, antihistamine nasal spray, or even surgery when there is a significant but correctable obstruction (such as a deviated septum or nasal polyps).
- **Using certain dental appliances** that sometimes help position the jaw in a way to relieve the obstruction.
- **Surgery to shrink or remove excessive soft tissue in the mouth and throat.** Occasionally other types of surgery, such as removal of large nasal polyps or correction of a congenital facial deformity, may be appropriate. For most people with sleep apnea, it is wise to try other approaches before resorting to a surgical solution. In children, on the other hand, removal of large tonsils and/or adenoids that are interfering with breathing at night may be more appropriate as a first step.

NARCOLEPSY

Narcolepsy is a disorder involving almost irresistible "sleep attacks" that can last from a few seconds to more than thirty minutes at a time. Narcolepsy seems to affect the part of the brain that regulates sleep and wakefulness, resulting in the sudden onset of REM sleep during the day, even when a person has had a normal amount of sleep the night before. The sleep attack may be preceded by hallucinations and can be embarrassing—when a person suddenly falls asleep during a social occasion or a class at school, for example—or dangerous, should it occur while one is driving or operating power equipment. Symptoms of narcolepsy commonly begin between puberty and the midtwenties and may be difficult to diagnose. Narcolepsy is associated with a phenomenon called cataplexy, in which a person suddenly loses muscle control and falls to the ground. Cataplexy can be brought on by strong emotions such as anger, laughter, or surprise. If all of these weren't irritating enough, people with narcolepsy may also experience sleep paralysis, brief periods when they are unable to move or speak while falling asleep or awakening.

People with narcolepsy should generally avoid night-shift work, irregular bedtimes, heavy meals, or alcohol intake. Once narcolepsy is diagnosed, a number of medications are available to manage these episodes, including stimulants to increase alertness, antidepressants (which help control the other phenomena associated with sleep attacks), and a newer drug called Provigil, which also improves alertness but without the other effects of stimulants.

PARASOMNIAS

A simple definition of a parasomnia is an unusual (even bizarre) or disturbing behavior occurring during sleep. The more formal definition is a disorder of sleep characterized by unwanted motor, verbal, or experiential phenomena associated with certain sleep stages or transitions.

At one time or another we have all experienced nightmares—frightening or unpleasant dreams that disrupt sleep. They are more common among the young than among adults, occurring in 35 to 45 percent of children between the ages of two and eighteen. Nightmares occur during REM sleep and are more common later in the sleep period. The dreams usually involve some sort of danger or threat. Upon awakening, the person having the nightmare is usually alert and aware of the present surroundings. Nightmares can be brought on by fever, illness, or certain medications but may also be related to stress or some other physically or psychologically traumatic event.

Night terrors involve the sudden awakening from an early phase of deep sleep with physical behavior associated with fright and intense fear, including screaming, thrashing, jabbering, and even fighting with whomever enters the room. Night terrors occur in 2 to 4 percent of young children and do not commonly continue into adulthood. (When they occur in adults, they may be difficult to distinguish from agitated sleepwalking.)

Sleepwalking, like night terrors, is probably a malfunction of the deeper phases of non-REM sleep. It occurs more commonly in childhood—the peak age is between four and eight—although if it persists into adolescence or adulthood, sleepwalking can be more dangerous. Episodes tend to occur earlier rather than later in the night. A glassy-eyed sleepwalker may wander aimlessly, carry objects around the house, get something to eat, urinate in an unusual location, go outside, and (when older) even attempt to drive. In children, no intervention is really needed other than to protect the sleepwalker from injury. A frequent sleepwalker may need additional safeguards, such as locking windows and doors and placing an alarm on the bedroom door. Sleepwalking adults who have had an injury (or a narrow escape) may be candidates for a bedtime medication that can effectively limit the number of episodes, or stop them altogether.

Sleep talking is a vocalization at night, which may range from a few words of nonsense to entire speeches. It is a harmless and usually temporary phenomenon, although it may startle or even frighten others within earshot. Sleep talking is sometimes associated with stress or an illness but does not need specific treatment.

Episodes of REM movement disorder (or REM sleep behavior disorder) resemble sleepwalking run amok. These are, in fact, very different events. Remember that during REM sleep the brain is very active generating dreams, but paradoxically (and for our safety) the body is virtually paralyzed. (REM sleep is, in fact, also called active sleep because so much is going on in the brain and paradoxical sleep because muscles are so quiet at the same time.) REM movement disorder demonstrates why this is so important. A person with this problem literally acts out his dreams, which unfortunately are not usually peaceful. Instead, the typical dreams involved in REM movement disorder seem to have been dialed in by a hyped-up video-game programmer. They are intense, full of action, often violent, and their dreamer may respond not merely with walking and talking, but with yelling, punching, kicking, jumping out of bed, running around, and at times even injuring himself or others.

While REM movement disorder may affect men or women at any age, more than 85 percent of people with this problem are men over fifty. Usually the person's temperament while awake in no way resembles the wild behavior that occurs during these episodes. Unfortunately, at least half of the people with this problem have other neurological disorders, such as Parkinson's disease, narcolepsy, or stroke. In fact, REM movement disorder may be the first manifestation of a different neurological disease that may not become apparent for months or even years. However, once the correct diagnosis has been made, both the sleep disturbance and its unruly manifestations can usually be controlled effectively with bedtime medications.

DELAYED SLEEP PHASE SYNDROME

Adolescence is likely to be the time in which delayed sleep phase syndrome (or DSPS) first occurs. Sometimes known as the "night owl syndrome," DSPS involves a shift in the circadian rhythm such that the affected person has difficulty falling asleep any earlier than from midnight to 3 A.M. He or she then has great difficulty awakening in the early morning. If allowed to sleep seven or eight hours, the person with DSPS feels perfectly refreshed and ready to work. For many self-employed individuals—especially those who write or do computer work and find evening hours less distracting—this schedule may not pose any problem. Unfortunately, classes or workdays frequently start at 8 or 9 A.M.—well before the night owl is ready to get up. As many as 7 percent of the general population may have DSPS, and some research suggests that it is more than twice as common among college students.[2]

If it is truly disrupting school and work performance, DSPS should not be ignored or written off as simple laziness. Sleeping medications are generally not effective in helping the person with DSPS fall asleep earlier in the evening, although melatonin has been found helpful for some. Exposure to bright light for thirty to sixty minutes after awakening early in the morning (typically between 6 and 8 A.M.) may help reset the internal clock. Light boxes that emit a standardized amount of white light are available commercially for this purpose. Because night owls usually find it easier to stay up later than to go to bed earlier, another approach called chronotherapy can help many with DSPS. This involves going to bed three hours later each night over a week's time, essentially resynchronizing a person's circadian rhythm to the schedule necessary for optimal school and work performance. Once a new (earlier) wake-up time is established, it must be maintained in order to avoid a relapse into the old late-night routine. Sleep experts generally recommend consulting with a physician trained in sleep disorders before embarking on a week of chronotherapy.

chapter 7

WHAT CAUSES MY ONGOING FATIGUE?

While many people can solve their problems with fatigue by changing a sleep habit, addressing a sleep disrupter, or treating a sleep disorder, many more will not find an immediate or obvious solution to their exhaustion. If you have experienced fatigue for an extended period of time and cannot pinpoint a specific cause, you are not alone. The next few chapters will focus on prolonged and chronic fatigue, with a particular emphasis on tiredness for which there is no apparent medical diagnosis. We will also discuss chronic fatigue syndrome (CFS), which is a severe form of fatigue defined by several specific criteria.

The Centers for Disease Control and Prevention (CDC) defines prolonged fatigue as persistent fatigue lasting one month or more, while chronic fatigue is defined as persistent or relapsing fatigue of six or more consecutive months. Both acute and chronic fatigue can have a host of physical, emotional, and even spiritual causes. More than one of these may be present in a given individual at the same time, and not all may be recognized by the person who feels tired. We can group them into a few basic categories:

1. **Physical fatigue caused by disease.** This is the type most readily identifiable by a doctor. It may be acute (such as the malaise of a flu) or chronic (such as the draining effects of a widespread cancer). If a medical disease is not readily apparent from a health history and physical exam, only in a small percentage of cases will additional studies (such as X rays and laboratory tests) reveal an unexpected physical disorder. Chronic fatigue syndrome (CFS) appears to fit in this category, although the exact nature of the physical disturbance remains unclear. We will look more closely at chronic fatigue syndrome in chapter 9 and discuss some other important medical causes for fatigue in chapter 8.

2. **Habits and lifestyle.** Poor physical conditioning, erratic eating patterns, obesity, stress, disrupted sleep, the use (or abuse) of certain prescription and nonprescription drugs, tobacco use, and excessive alcohol intake can all contribute to tiredness. While these issues cannot be resolved overnight, addressing them over time can definitely improve energy.

3. **Acute mental and emotional fatigue.** This is usually tied to a specific event: working on a difficult homework assignment, preparing tax returns, packing for a long trip, hosting a large family gathering,

and so forth. Many of these situations and the tiredness they create have a limited impact and duration (typically a few days or perhaps weeks). More serious events such as the sudden death of a loved one, a business reversal, or a divorce will have both immediate and long-lasting repercussions that can contribute to fatigue that lasts for months or years.

4. **Chronic mental and emotional fatigue.** Long-term conflict or dissatisfaction with relationships, work, and the circumstances of everyday life can be stressful and draining. Ongoing responsibility for elderly parents or for a spouse or other loved one with failing health, a significant disability, dementia, or other chronic problems can be a setup for fatigue. Very often someone with this type of fatigue is fighting battles on more than one front: Pressure all day on the job may be followed by ongoing conflict at home, for example.

5. **Depression.** Frequently the primary cause of ongoing fatigue, depression may be reactive (related to outside circumstances), endogenous (related to biochemical processes in the brain), or a mix of both. Depression may be acute, chronic, or recurrent. Very often a person visiting a physician's office to address fatigue may not be aware of a mood problem, although often those who live and work with him or her have noticed it. Needless to say, it is important that depression be considered during an evaluation

for fatigue, as many tired people feel considerably better after they are treated appropriately for this problem. Other mood and thought disturbances, such as bipolar disorder, schizophrenia, and eating disorders (anorexia nervosa and bulimia nervosa), may be associated with fatigue as well.

6. **Spiritual and moral issues.** These can't be detected through a physical exam or laboratory tests, but they may play a role in causing fatigue. A person who has a vibrant relationship with God and who senses His loving presence on a daily basis has a reason to feel optimistic and energetic even when other factors that might generate fatigue (such as a physical illness) are present. It should be noted, however, that spiritual health does not guarantee freedom from physical or even emotional disturbances—including fatigue. At the same time, one who feels estranged from God, who consciously behaves in ways that violate God's standards, or who believes that there is no God and that life is pointless may eventually experience a melancholy that can only be relieved by establishing or restoring a relationship with his Creator. Spiritual malaise may also be a by-product of other types of fatigue. If we're tired for other reasons—or simply overcommitted—we may not feel we have the energy or time to connect with God on our own or to gather with others for that purpose. God may seem distant, detached, or even absent.

SOME CHARACTERISTICS OF CHRONIC FATIGUE

People who are chronically tired usually spend a fair number of waking hours (or sleepless nights) thinking about possible causes and remedies for their problem. Some come up with reasonable ideas, many more remain perplexed, and a few arrive at far-fetched conclusions. In order to gain some perspective on this problem, it is helpful to understand some basic principles that apply to most cases of chronic fatigue.

Fatigue, like pain, is subjective. Fatigue is a symptom that one can feel and describe. It is not a physical characteristic, such as heart rate or blood sugar, that can be measured. More importantly, fatigue is usually drastically influenced by one's emotional state, and especially by expectations for the immediate future. If you're feeling lethargic at work in the middle of the afternoon, an unexpected call from the president of the company will most likely spring you to life in a matter of seconds. Mild symptoms of fatigue may be ignored when circumstances are enjoyable and interesting, but they become a ball and chain in the face of an unpleasant task. It may take a crowbar to get children out of bed on a typical school morning, but watch the miraculous burst of activity when they suddenly realize that it's snowing and school has been canceled.

Chronic fatigue often has more than one cause. Occasionally a single medical problem (for example, anemia caused by iron deficiency) is the cause of ongoing tiredness. More often, fatigue is like a river fed by several streams. Several years of consuming more calories than needed every day may have created a physical burden of twenty, fifty, or one hundred extra pounds. There may be ongoing frustration at work. The daily round of chores at home may feel like an endless treadmill. A stack of bills may overwhelm the paycheck. A relationship with one's spouse or children may be in constant turmoil. And a medical problem may be lurking behind the scenes. Defining the problems and mapping these various "streams" can be a major challenge. Yet identifying causes is only the beginning.

Chronic fatigue infrequently has a single, "magic bullet" cure. The person who comes to a physician asking for "something to pep me up" will usually walk away disappointed, especially if the practitioner takes a careful and methodical approach to evaluating the cause of fatigue. There is, however, no shortage of supplements, potions, diets, and eccentric therapies that are promoted as surefire energy boosters. Some people find that these approaches seem to improve matters for a while, often for reasons that make little or no sense biologically. This may happen because the tired person feels energized by the belief that someone has found an answer to this problem, no matter how far-fetched the "cure" may be. Unfortunately, this apparent solution may divert attention from more important issues, such as lack of exercise or excessive weight.

Paradoxically, in most cases managing chronic fatigue requires *effort* by the individual who is tired. This is especially true when lifestyle changes, such as exercise and weight loss, are needed. While many who are chronically fatigued may feel too tired to do what is needed to reduce their tiredness, there are in fact few passive cures for this problem. What is done *to* us or *for* us tends to be less effective in raising energy levels on a lasting basis than what is done *by* us.

Raising one's energy level is usually a slow process. This should come as no surprise, given the multitude of factors that may contribute to chronic fatigue, the shortage of effective magic bullets, and the need to expend some effort and make changes if we are to improve how we feel. Most chronically tired people cannot say exactly when their weariness started, and few can identify exactly when things begin to turn around. Managing this problem is like steering an ocean liner. It usually requires a number of small course corrections that result in a change in position some time later.

chapter 8

WHEN SHOULD I CONSULT A DOCTOR?

In general, it is important to be evaluated medically for significant fatigue lasting more than two or three weeks, unless there is a cause that will eventually resolve on its own (for example, lack of sleep caused by a fussy newborn in the house). In addition, certain symptoms indicate the need for a medical evaluation *sooner* rather than later:

- fever over 100°
- unusual sweating, especially during the night
- significant headache, especially if it is new, persistent, or unusual
- light-headedness or overt fainting episodes
- shortness of breath
- persistent or recurring pain, especially in the chest or abdomen
- nausea and vomiting
- jaundice (a yellow-orange color of skin)
- persistent diarrhea
- dark or bloody bowel movements
- painful, frequent, or difficult passage of urine
- blood in the urine, with or without pain

- painful or swollen joints
- pain or swelling in the legs
- intolerance of heat or cold
- change in menstrual flow, whether increased, decreased, or absent
- unexplained weight loss

Keep in mind that these symptoms may or may not be related to the cause of fatigue—indeed, they may or may not even indicate the presence of a significant medical condition. Shortness of breath, for example, may result from anxiety, congestive heart failure, or a number of other problems. Each of these symptoms may be associated with fatigue, and all of them must be addressed, though in different ways.

HELPING YOUR DOCTOR TRACK DOWN YOUR FATIGUE PROBLEM

If you are going to seek help from your physician about fatigue, make an appointment specifically to address that question. Don't ask "Why am I so tired all the time?" at the end of a visit for another problem, because it is impossible to address this concern appropriately in a few minutes. In addition, you will get a lot more accomplished if you are prepared to offer specific details about your fatigue. A complaint such as "I can't sleep" or "I'm always tired" is a starting place, but your doctor needs much more information than that.

Before your appointment, be prepared for your

health-care provider to ask the following questions. (You may want to record them in your diary.)

How long have you been tired, and did your fatigue problem begin suddenly or gradually? If you feel as if you've been tired for years, these questions may be hard to answer, but the more specific you can be, the better. When the time frame is uncertain, it sometimes helps to consider the last time you truly felt well. If fatigue began recently (within the past several weeks), or you can state specifically when the trouble started ("I felt great until June 15"), an identifiable medical problem is more likely. If the answer is "I can't remember when I really felt well," you should be open to the possibility that ongoing mood and lifestyle issues need to be addressed.

Does the fatigue interfere with any daily activities? Have you canceled any plans because of fatigue? Many people *feel* tired even while they remain very active and productive. (In fact, their fatigue may be related to overcommitment.) Some, however, are so pro-foundly affected by tiredness that work, recreation, and even the basic functions of life may be disrupted. In this case, certain diagnoses should be ruled out by a careful medical evaluation. Significant depression can cause a person to withdraw from normal activities. By definition, chronic fatigue syndrome (CFS) is tiredness that signifi-cantly limits a person's ability to function at work or home.

When your fatigue began, was it accompanied by any other symptoms? Symptoms that occurred at the onset of the fatigue problem (or perhaps preceded it) may provide important clues about the cause. For example, a combination of fever, aches, loss of appetite, and headache followed by prolonged tiredness usually suggests that a virus started the problem and left fatigue in its wake. Another example: The passage of one or more very dark stools followed by ongoing fatigue could signal blood loss in the intestine and a resulting anemia.

Are specific physical symptoms accompanying the fatigue now? Symptoms that accompany fatigue on a long-term basis can suggest directions to explore. Some—fever, unexplained weight loss, and the others listed on pages 53–54—may indicate the presence of a specific disease and require further medical evaluation. Symptoms such as insomnia, poor concentration, dizziness, and numbness or tingling that migrate all over the body may also point to specific illness, but often they are related to mood disturbances such as anxiety and depression. (When physical symptoms and mood problems mix, it can be difficult to determine which is the cause and which is the effect.) As with fatigue, it will help the physician if you can offer specific characteristics of these other symptoms (e.g., How long have they been present? What, if anything, makes them better or worse? Have they ever happened before?). If you have a number of complaints, don't be disappointed if all of them are not addressed fully in one sitting.

Is fatigue relieved by a good night's sleep? Do you have any trouble falling or staying asleep? The relationship of fatigue to sleep is an important one. If tiredness stems from an overabundance of activities and a shortage of hours left for sleeping, an extra couple of hours one night or a weekend of "catch-up" sleep can work wonders. On the other hand, chronically tired people often complain that they feel no better when waking in the morning than they did when crawling under the covers. Disturbed sleep—whether difficulty falling asleep, waking early, a strong desire to sleep both night and day, or a combination of these—is also an important issue for the depressed person, who almost invariably complains of chronic fatigue.

It may be helpful to keep a simple diary for a few days. In the morning, write down when you went to bed, when you got up, and estimates of how long it took to fall asleep, how many times you were awake (include how long you were awake and whether anything specific awakened you), and how many hours of sleep you got. In the evening, note how you felt during the day and the time and length of any nap(s) you took.

Is the fatigue problem actually chronic drowsiness? Do you fight sleepiness during the day (especially when sitting quietly or while driving)? Do

you fall asleep right after dinner or as soon as your head hits the pillow? Has anyone noticed that you snore or have erratic breathing patterns during the night? If the answer to one or more of these is yes, the problem may be a sleep disorder—especially sleep apnea, which is often associated with snoring. Because they interfere with the normal restorative effects of sleep, these disorders can cause a person to feel drowsy even after seven or eight hours of sleep. Also, many of us become fatigued during the afternoon, often immediately after lunch or between 2 and 4 P.M. This is at least partly due to the normal phenomenon known as circadian rhythm, which can cause a dip in energy and increased sleepiness during this time frame. Sleep disorders and the circadian rhythm are reviewed in more detail in chapter 6.

Does fatigue improve on weekends and vacations? Do you go to bed and get up at different times on weekends and vacations? If your fatigue disappears at 5 P.M. every Friday or evaporates on the beach at Maui, chances are you have some issues related to the responsibilities of the workweek. On the other hand, if weariness interferes with or aborts an activity you normally relish, a medical problem or a significant depression is more likely.

Are there any major stresses or changes in your life at this time? Challenging life situations often have physical effects, including inability to sleep and lack of energy. We address some specific lifestyle energy drainers in chapter 11, "How Can I Feel More Energized?"

Are you taking any medications (prescription or nonprescription) or supplements? Sedation and fatigue are common side effects of a number of prescription and over-the-counter drugs, which can contribute to chronic fatigue. Occasionally a medication that normally does not cause fatigue may prove to be a major energy drainer for a particular individual. In some cases, a medication review may uncover a chain reaction leading to fatigue. For example, the chronic use of an anti-inflammatory drug to treat arthritis might cause ongoing blood loss into the intestine, which in turn could eventually lead to a tiring iron-deficiency anemia.

Even if one or more medications may be contributing to chronic fatigue, it is important *not* to change dosage (or stop taking a drug) before checking with your physician. Furthermore, if possible it's wise not to make more than one change at a time in an established medication regime, because the results can be confusing. If you feel better (or worse) after making multiple changes, it will be hard to tell which is responsible. Finally, be careful not to assume there's a relationship between symptoms (especially fatigue) and medications. Some people assume that if they're not feeling well, whatever was prescribed most recently must be the culprit—especially if they weren't too excited about taking it in the first place.

WHAT TYPES OF MEDICATIONS CAN BE ASSOCIATED WITH CHRONIC FATIGUE?

Antihistamines. The older (sometimes called first generation) forms of these common remedies for colds and allergies can cause immediate drowsiness or ongoing fatigue when taken on a daily basis. Newer antihistamines are far less likely to cause drowsiness or fatigue.

Drugs that lower blood pressure (antihypertensives). Certain beta blockers, which slow the heart rate and decrease the forcefulness of each contraction, can cause fatigue. Fortunately, the blood pressure medications that are most widely used today usually do *not* cause fatigue. These include the diuretics (or water pills) that decrease the body's fluid volume, the angiotensin converting enzyme inhibitors (more commonly called ACE inhibitors), the angiotensin receptor blockers (or ARBs), the calcium channel blockers, and the alpha blockers.

Even a drug that normally causes no (or minimal) side effects may cause some individuals to feel tired. If this seems to be occurring, some careful trial and error should be carried out under the supervision of one's physician. One important reminder: Some people who have had hypertension for a long time, especially the elderly, may feel fatigued with a lower blood pressure—at least for a while. Therefore, it is not a good idea to give up on a medication until enough time has passed to assess its various effects.

Antidepressants. Ironically, these are often the medications prescribed to treat chronic fatigue caused by depression. The right agent in the right patient can produce a dramatic improvement, but individual responses vary. For some people these drugs can be sedating, particularly during the first few days. As with blood pressure medications, it is wise not to discontinue one of these drugs too quickly, since side effects are often temporary and benefits may not be noticed for a few weeks.

Anxiety-reducing medications (anxiolytics). The drugs most widely used to reduce anxiety are the benzodiazepines. They are by definition sedating and thus can produce fatigue. In some people this occurs because these medications relieve nervousness that accompanies depression, but not depression itself, making other symptoms (including fatigue) more apparent. For others, severe anxiety itself drains energy, and so one of these medications can improve both anxiety and fatigue—at least for a while. Unfortunately, long-term use can result in both psychological and physical dependence. If you take one of these drugs regularly and feel tired, a discussion with your physician is definitely in order.

Medications used for epilepsy, Parkinson's disease, and Alzheimer's disease. Treating these illnesses requires careful monitoring of the benefits and side effects of medications, although often these can be alleviated or prevented by using newer agents, tracking blood levels, and adjusting dosing schedules. An important caution: *Under no circumstance should any treatment for epilepsy be changed without consulting the prescribing physician.* The most common cause of an unexpected seizure is reducing or stopping medication.

Pain relievers in the opiate class. These medications are inherently sedating. When they are taken chronically, this effect becomes less noticeable because the body becomes habituated, or accustomed, to the drug.

Anyone who takes prescription pain medications for a prolonged period may feel fatigued for other reasons. Chronic pain syndromes are draining and frequently associated with depression. Addressing the pain problem (and finding the most appropriate medications to help manage it) usually is a multidisciplinary task, which may require help from a primary-care physician, a pain specialist, a counselor, and a psychiatrist, among others. Frequently a team approach, such as is used in pain clinics associated with medical centers and university hospitals, is most appropriate.

Drugs used to treat certain intestinal disorders. These drugs also can cause fatigue, although not many are taken on an ongoing basis. Some medications for nausea and seasickness are inherently sedating, but fortunately these are rarely needed for long periods of time. (Other less sedating options are also available.) Metoclopramide (Reglan), once prescribed widely for heartburn and still used for certain types of ongoing intestinal problems, can cause fatigue in some people. Antispasmodics used to treat the cramps of irritable bowel syndrome can be sedating.

WHAT MEDICAL CONDITIONS CAN BE ASSOCIATED WITH FATIGUE?

This list of medical problems that are often associated with prolonged and chronic fatigue is not intended to alarm you, but rather to give you a feel for the breadth of conditions that your physician might consider when addressing this symptom.

- Chronic failure of one or more vital organs: heart, lungs, liver, or kidneys
- Infection, such as acute infectious mononucleosis, influenza, HIV/AIDS, hepatitis, tuberculosis, Lyme disease, and chronic sinusitis
- Anemia (an abnormally low red blood cell count), which may have a number of possible causes
- Neoplasm, a benign or malignant (cancerous) growth, including uncontrolled proliferation of certain types of blood cells (such as leukemia) or lymph tissue (lymphoma)
- Endocrine (hormonal) disturbances, including abnormally high or low levels of thyroid hormone, diabetes (especially when blood glucose is markedly elevated), abnormalities of adrenal gland function (which are quite rare), menopause, or in men, low testosterone levels
- Autoimmune (often called rheumatologic) syndromes, such as rheumatoid arthritis, systemic lupus erythema-

tosus, Sjögren's syndrome, dermatomyositis, and thyroiditis, that occur when the immune system inappropriately inflames and damages the body's own tissues

- Neurological disorders, including multiple sclerosis and Parkinson's disease
- Heavy metal exposure and toxicity, such as lead poisoning
- Chronic pain problems that provoke both physical and emotional fatigue as well as depression, or that are controlled by medications that contribute to fatigue

TWO NONDIAGNOSES FOR CHRONIC FATIGUE

The frequent failure to find a clear-cut diagnosis for chronic fatigue has, not surprisingly, led to a number of theories about its cause that have not passed scientific scrutiny. Two that continue to circulate in books, Web sites, and other media are hypoglycemia and chronic candidiasis.

For decades, hypoglycemia or low blood glucose (also referred to as low blood sugar) has been blamed for causing chronic fatigue and numerous other symptoms. For many reasons it is an unlikely suspect for causing long-term fatigue. The most compelling of these is that our body is engineered to ensure that any drop in blood glucose level will be transient rather than chronic. Even if a person's blood sugar drops far enough to cause fatigue or other symptoms, the body's response (or the next meal, snack, or glass of juice) will raise it relatively quickly. (The exception would be a profound hypoglycemia caused by an excessive dose of insulin or other glucose-lowering medication taken by a person with diabetes. In that case, however, emergency medical care would be necessary to correct the problem.) Bottom line: Even if a person experiences brief periods of hypoglycemia for whatever reason, these would not be expected to cause chronic fatigue.

Chronic candidiasis has been blamed for many problems but lacks scientific credibility. The yeast species *Candida albicans* is best known for growing in places that are wet and warm: skin folds, the vagina, and occasionally the mouth, where the infection is called thrush. It can also trouble diabetics and those on prolonged or intensive antibiotics. Its common infections produce local irritation and usually respond to medications applied directly to the affected area. In a small number of people with immune deficiencies (such as cancer patients receiving chemotherapy or AIDS patients), *Candida* can spread throughout the body, causing a devastating illness.

The term *candidiasis hypersensitivity syndrome* refers to a constellation of symptoms, encompassing nearly every organ system, that are said to arise from disturbed immune function caused by excessive growth of *Candida albicans*. The diagnosis is not based on any specific test but rather on the individual's history.

Common treatments include a special diet (that among other things avoids "all foods containing yeast and mold," said to encourage the growth of *Candida*), plus nutritional supplements and possibly antifungal medications.

Unfortunately, the symptoms of candidiasis hypersensitivity syndrome are so numerous that nearly everyone may experience at least one or two at any given time. There is no specific test that identifies it, but only an assumption that the diagnosis is confirmed if a person feels better in response to the proposed therapies. Furthermore, this concept lacks a credible explanation of the mechanism by which *Candida albicans* might produce so many generalized symptoms, or how the treatments (other than the antifungal agents) might have any impact on this process. The bottom line: The promoters of candidiasis hypersensitivity syndrome have yet to present convincing evidence for their claim that chronic fatigue (and numerous other everyday ailments) is caused by this common organism.

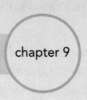
DO I HAVE CHRONIC
FATIGUE SYNDROME?

Sometimes if fatigue is severe and prolonged and other tests are normal, the diagnosis of chronic fatigue syndrome (CFS) may be considered. Chronic fatigue syndrome is, fortunately, *not* the diagnosis for the vast majority of people who feel tired on an ongoing basis. According to the case definition (revised in 1994) from the Centers for Disease Control and Prevention:

> Chronic fatigue syndrome is a debilitating and complex disorder characterized by profound fatigue that is not improved by bed rest and that may be worsened by physical or mental activity. Persons with CFS most often function at a substantially lower level of activity than they were capable of before the onset of illness. In addition to these key defining characteristics, patients report various nonspecific symptoms, including weakness, muscle pain, impaired memory and/or mental concentration, insomnia, and post-exertional fatigue lasting more than 24 hours. In some cases, CFS can persist for years.[3]

A typical early presentation of CFS might be fatigue that lasts weeks or months and is not relieved by a few restful days and nights of good sleep. The onset of CFS may appear to follow an otherwise innocuous infection or illness such as a cold, bronchitis, or a stomach virus. For some it may follow a bout of infectious mononucleosis (the familiar "mono" most often seen among teenagers and young adults), or it may begin after a period of unusual stress or high workload. For many people with CFS, symptoms develop gradually, with no obvious illness or precipitating event.

DIAGNOSING CHRONIC FATIGUE SYNDROME

CFS is defined by a number of key symptoms and an *absence* of specific physical, laboratory, or other diagnostic findings that would point toward a different diagnosis. According to the CDC, a case of CFS is defined as persistent or relapsing chronic fatigue with the following features:

- The feeling of exhaustion is either new or had a definite onset sometime in the past (as opposed to being lifelong). The person who says "I've been tired ever since I can remember" does not have CFS.
- It is not the result of ongoing exertion and is not substantially relieved by rest.
- It results in a significant reduction in activity that may impact job, home, school, or social life, or all of these areas.

• It is not explained by some other medical or psychiatric diagnosis after an appropriate and thorough clinical evaluation. Note that one cannot self-diagnose CFS, because the diagnosis requires that an appropriate medical evaluation to rule out other causes of fatigue has been carried out.

The diagnosis of CFS requires that fatigue as described above has been present for six or more consecutive months and that at least four of the following (known as primary symptoms) have also been present during the same time frame:

• Impairment in short-term memory or concentration that is significant enough to cause a substantial reduction in activities affecting home, work, school, and social life
• Sore throat
• Tender lymph nodes
• Muscle pain
• Pain in multiple joints, but without swelling or redness
• Headache of a new type, pattern, or severity
• Unrefreshing sleep
• Malaise lasting more than twenty-four hours after exertion

Other symptoms may be present in addition to these.

A person who is suffering from severe ongoing fatigue should undergo a thorough medical evaluation. This should include a comprehensive history and physical examination, including a review of all medications and supplements in past and current use. A basic mental status examination should be done to identify any abnormalities in mood, intellectual function, memory, and personality. In addition, a battery of basic laboratory screening tests should be done including a complete blood count, a panel of metabolic blood chemistries, thyroid functions, urinalysis, and a marker for inflammation known as the erythrocyte sedimentation rate ("sed rate" for short). Any abnormal result revealed by this evaluation must be pursued, and other tests may be indicated as well, depending on the individual clinical situation and presentation.

It is important to note that at present no tests can *prove* someone has chronic fatigue syndrome. This being the case, it should come as no surprise that a reliable and effective treatment for this disorder has yet to be found. (Unproven treatment options, on the other hand, are abundant.)

CFS, therefore, is a problem that is managed rather than cured. A combination of measures, including a sleep evaluation, medication, a carefully structured exercise program, and counseling, are often recommended by physicians to help patients cope with this disorder.[4]

chapter 10

WHAT CAN I DO ABOUT CHRONIC TIREDNESS?

In the majority of cases, a medical examination will not reveal a precise explanation for a patient's fatigue. Those who leave their doctors' offices without a specific, treatable diagnosis may or may not be given ideas to help resolve the fatigue, depending on the expectations of the patient and the inclinations of the doctor. Everyday medical practice is so demanding that even the most caring physician may be hard-pressed to look very far beyond medical problems into other causes of chronic fatigue, which may involve important conflicts at home or work, mood disturbances such as depression and anxiety, personal habits and lifestyle, and spiritual problems.

Even if your doctor hasn't come up with a diagnosis, don't lose heart or give up. There are a number of steps that you can take to address your fatigue. All of the suggestions that follow will be helpful, regardless of the cause of the fatigue.

Get regular exercise. People who exercise regularly and are fit are less likely to struggle with fatigue. Even if you feel too tired to make the effort, regular physical activity—even a modest amount that you gradually increase every day—is one of the few measures that will reliably improve chronic fatigue.

Deal with excess weight. The more overweight a person becomes, the more likely he is to develop physical problems that contribute to fatigue.

Take a careful look at your mood. As we mentioned already, ongoing anxiety and depression are among the most common and treatable causes of chronic fatigue. Assessing these conditions may require a visit with your physician, a qualified counselor, or both.

Take a careful inventory of the quality of your relationships. Ongoing conflict at home, work, or school can be a major energy drainer in your life. If you experience constant turmoil with your spouse, children, or parents or are having difficulty developing a network of supportive friends, an honest and open discussion with a counselor or your pastor is in order. We will look at the problem of ongoing conflict at home in chapter 11 (beginning on page 87).

Evaluate your relationship with God and your purpose in life. Do you feel stuck in a routine? What motivates you to get out of bed every morning? Do you have any goals, spiritual or otherwise? Lacking a worthwhile purpose or pursuing possessions and pleasures that ultimately amount to a "chasing after the wind" (as described by King Solomon in the book of Ecclesiastes) will eventually bring a person to a state of weariness and even despair. Even a cursory reading of the Bible makes it clear that God does not suffer from chronic fatigue and that those who are empowered by His Spirit to accomplish His purposes manifest remarkable energy. (See the book of Acts in the New Testament for some noteworthy examples.) If your spiritual life is dead in the water or has never been launched in the first place, we encourage you to meet with your pastor or become involved in a church that is manifesting life, love, and growth.

chapter 11

HOW CAN
I FEEL MORE ENERGIZED?

Addressing Nine Potential Lifestyle Energy Drainers

Whether or not you are dealing with medical illness, depression, spiritual dryness, or turbulent relationships, the following nine issues can affect anyone. They are important enough to examine a little more closely.

1. **Overcommitment: too many irons in the fire.** Do you ever attempt to set a date for a night out with your spouse or close friends and find nothing available in your schedule for three weeks? Do you feel like your life consists of an unending series of brushfires, with the hottest and the closest flames getting the most attention? Do you often get the sinking feeling that you're doing a half-baked job on a number of projects rather than an excellent job on a few?

   If you answered yes to one or more of these questions and feel perpetually tired, begin the challenging (and often lengthy) task of dealing with your cluttered calendar. Remember that you must do this prayerfully and carefully. You may not be able to disengage from ongoing commitments without giving plenty of advance notice and perhaps assisting in passing the baton to someone else. If you are married, involve your spouse in these discussions. Whether you're married or single, you may want to ask one or more trustworthy friends to hold you accountable to this de-commitment process.

2. **Undercommitment: too few meaningful activities.** In contrast to the overcommitted, some people attend only to the most basic needs of life. They are stifled and usually tired because they lack the energizing purposes and goals that would take them beyond the four walls of home. This is a particular risk for those who find themselves adrift after retirement. Having a compelling purpose for your life is energizing, and the good news is that there are unlimited opportunities to make a difference in the lives of other people. Consider what might be your purpose beyond attending to everyday routines. There is no shortage of worthwhile projects in your own church, a local hospital or nursing home, the neighborhood, or even in some distant country. What skills do you have that could assist someone

else? Can you teach a disadvantaged person something you know—perhaps how to read or how to balance a checkbook? You may change his or her life. Is there a nursing home in town? Many who are confined there would be overjoyed to have a regular visitor.

Does your community have a crisis pregnancy center? These ministries, which provide practical assistance to women, are always in need of volunteers for all sorts of projects. (They may also be called a pregnancy resource center, pregnancy care center, or women's resource center.) Your church may already be involved with a center, or you can check with umbrella organizations such as Care Net, which you can reach at (703) 478-5661 or http://www.care-net.org, or Heartbeat International, (888) 550-7577 or http://www.heartbeatinternational.org.

Is there a prison or jail nearby? Prison Fellowship can put you to work in all sorts of significant activities that make a decisive difference in inmates' lives. For information about local projects, contact Prison Fellowship at (877) 478-0100 or online at http://www.pfm.org. If you help change the world for even one or two people, you'll feel better as well.

3. **Clutter: the accumulated stuff of life.** When we combine our all-too-human urge to acquire things

with a reluctance to let go of them, our gradual accumulation of possessions can become an indoor overgrowth of weeds that will suffocate us unless it is periodically pruned. A home or apartment crammed from one end to the other with "treasures" can be a major energy drainer.

Decluttering can be a step toward tranquility and an energizing experience, especially if you turn on some upbeat music while tossing out junk that will never be missed. Limit yourself to one room or closet per session to avoid feeling overwhelmed. Has an article of clothing not been donned for a year or more? Goodwill will find it a nice home. Have you looked at those magazines from last year? You won't this year either. Do you need to keep every piece of artwork Johnny brings home from pre-school? Unless you want to be buried alive by the time he reaches junior high, pick the best of the lot, preserve them carefully and faithfully, and toss the rest. What about the old videocassettes of shows you recorded years ago for viewing at some later date? You can probably rent most of them at the video store any day of the week (assuming they're worth watching). And so on. Once some order is restored in your home or workplace, notice how good you feel. To maintain that positive emotion, remember that the "round file" can be one of your best friends.

4. **Debt: the paper chain.** Financial bondage can be a component of an overcommitted and frantic lifestyle—one that we would call "marginless"—and a contributor to emotional distress. Significant debt and pressing financial obligations can also be an enormous energy drain. Getting out from under a serious burden of debt requires an approach similar to that needed to lose weight. We need to face the reality that there are more things to buy than we can afford, and we need to get a grip on the flow of our own income and expenses. We then need to develop a plan that we can live with for a long time, and stay with it. More than one financial planner has suggested taking the smallest debt first and paying it off while maintaining the minimum requirements on the others. Each account sent to zero can be the occasion for a "retirement party." In addition, being accountable to someone else will help us maintain the chosen course when temptation is at hand. For help in this area, we recommend the resources of Crown Financial Ministries. Its ten-week small group study, which many churches offer on an ongoing basis, is particularly useful. For more information check http://www.crown.org on the Internet, call (800) 722-1976, or write to Crown Financial Ministries at P.O. Box 100, Gainesville, GA 30503-0100.

5. **Workaholism: breaking the commandment to rest.** This specific form of overcommitment can occur both in the corporate world and among the self-employed. The common denominator is a compulsion to attend to the job, the business, the clients, the patients, the project, or the store without reasonable boundaries on the number of hours in the day or the number of days in the week.

Hard-driving corporate types are actually not the worst violators of the fourth commandment. The self-employed, especially those with small businesses, are always vulnerable in this area. They frequently don't feel secure enough to forget about their enterprises for a day, so they carry work home in their mind (if not in their briefcase) after business hours and may deprive family members of the precious time and attention that they need. Second on the list for workaholic risk are caregivers: physicians, psychologists, social workers, and pastors. Since the dimensions of human need in any community are virtually limitless, those who meet needs for a living can easily burn out with exhaustion if they are always "on call."

Obviously diligence, responsibility, and excellence are noble goals for corporations and small businesses. Family enterprises can be meaningful for all concerned, and reaching out to those in need is a high calling. But there is always infinitely more work to do than can ever be done, and there are more needs within one city block than any of us can ever meet. Solid lines must be drawn in our life, across which work must not be given a toehold. The line may involve a *place* (such as home, unless the office is at home) or more importantly, a *time*. Here's the bottom line and the essence of God's commandment to rest on the Sabbath: *It is extremely important to have a minimum of one day per week—very often, but not always, Sunday—during which one's primary vocation is off-limits.* Those who fail to set aside this day over an extended period of time can count on being tired. When Jesus noted that the Sabbath was made for man and not man for the Sabbath (see Mark 2:23-28), He was talking about more than religious observances. God commanded a day off every week for the sake of the survival and sanity of the humans He loves.

Ideally, the day off is not the time to clean the garage or check off the first five items on a honey-do list. (Of course, for many people some physical effort exerted on behalf of one's home or garden can actually be diverting or even refreshing.) It should be a time to refresh, reflect, recreate, worship, and spend time with people we care about. Sometimes it is necessary to escape to a park, beach, zoo, movie, museum, or whatever puts distance between us and our vocational brushfires. Unfortunately, cell phones and pagers, as useful as they can be, can tether us to our work. One of life's most courageous and difficult decisions may be declining to answer calls during time that has been set aside for family or personal restoration.

6. **The TGIF syndrome: why work?** Pop quiz—(1) If you suddenly inherited a million dollars, would you keep working at your present job? (2) Does a cloud of gloom hang over your workplace (or your kitchen table) every Monday morning? Does it gradually lift as the week progresses? Obviously, the vast majority of us find it necessary to be gainfully employed. However, if your work generates no greater satisfaction than a paycheck every other week, you may spend five or six days each week fighting fatigue.

If you're not particularly enthusiastic about your job, reflect on what your work accomplishes. Who benefits from what you do? If the answer is no one in particular and if after careful assessment you decide that your work is essentially meaningless, think creatively about other ways to spend forty or more hours of work per week. On the other hand, before blowing off steam about "this lousy job" and making noises about quitting, some precautionary prayer and wise counsel are in order. Jumping from job to job may be symptomatic of a deeper lack of contentment or a permanently critical and ungrateful attitude. Furthermore, perhaps your workplace is an arena God has provided in which you are to be salt and light. There are usually plenty of needs to be met within a few feet of any desk or workbench. The apostle Paul did not consider his occupation as a tentmaker to be his primary mission in life—but he didn't belittle it either, since it gave him a certain level of independence as he pursued his goals of preaching and teaching.

7. **Raising small children: on call at all times.** Some of the most tired people who pass the portals of doctors' offices are the parents of infants and toddlers. Anyone who has assumed responsibility for young children for more than a few minutes understands that parenting them is one of the most demanding full-time tasks on earth. Bringing a newborn home is challenging even for a married couple who is well prepared, motivated, and supported by family and friends. The cry of a newborn baby is not a particularly pleasant sound, but it serves a vital purpose— it's a powerful stimulus for parents to feed, change, rock, and provide other necessary care frequently both day and night. When a baby cries on and on, especially during the night, even the most committed parents can begin to feel edgy and put-upon. For those in less favorable circumstances—single moms, young couples with very limited resources, or parents whose feelings about the child-rearing

process are mixed—the response to a combination of unending responsibility and chronic fatigue arising from sleepless nights may escalate into frustration, anger, and even child abuse or neglect.

After newborns and infants have graduated to toddler and preschooler status, staying at home with them may feel rewarding, exhausting, stimulating, and mind-numbing—sometimes all in the same day. What do you do when the kids have left the room and you're still watching *Sesame Street*? How many times can you hear the latest Barney CD before you start singing it—when no one else is around? What does it mean when the high point of your day is watching reruns of a twenty-year-old sitcom while the kids lie down for a nap? Why bother to clean up the house when it automatically returns to total disorder within thirty minutes? Is it possible to be attentive to the needs of small children without your brain turning to mush?

Lack of sleep, lack of adult conversation, and lack of any sense of forward motion (except watching the kids get bigger) drain vast amounts of energy from the most talented, motivated, and dedicated stay-at-home parents. In addition, and probably most importantly, lack of recognition for the job being done drives many stay-at-home parents into unnecessary despair, as they picture their friends advancing in what may appear to be glamorous (or at least more interesting) careers and wonder if they're foolish for staying home.

There are many ways to plug (or at least slow) this very important energy drain. If you are a parent who stays home, consider the following ideas.

- Develop some appropriate expectations for this season. This is a surprisingly brief passage, though it may seem like an eternity now. Life is not passing you by. There will be many years ahead to carve your niche in society, if that is what you are called to do.

- Remind yourself of the importance of this job, even if no one else seems to appreciate it. These years are significant for both you and the children, and being an eyewitness to your children's daily changes and growth can be fascinating.

- Keep learning. Who says the mind has to go numb for several years? What books do you want to read besides *Goodnight Moon* and *The Runaway Bunny*? What was your favorite course in high school or your major in college? No one said you couldn't keep exploring those topics or continue taking courses at a local college when the children get a little older.

- Cultivate relationships with other adults (of the same sex). Regularly scheduled times of grown-up conversation are critical, and your spouse may not be able to meet all of your needs in this area. (This is especially important for the single parent, who is bearing all of the responsibility single-handedly.)

- Find the best babysitters in the area, and reward them well (if you can). Doing so will allow you to have some time-outs on a regular basis—not for errands but for brief periods of personal refreshment. Going out with friends or having some time alone is both legitimate and necessary. When cash is short, a resourceful alternative is the babysitting co-op, an arrangement in which several people use a barter system to swap child care. If you are blessed with loving grandparents nearby, let them spoil the kids for a few hours (or even overnight) while you get a break.

• If you are a single parent, take strong measures to maintain your sanity and balance. You have some of the greatest challenges of all, since there may not be another adult in the vicinity to share child-rearing responsibilities with you. Don't be afraid to let your church family know about some of your needs, and be patient if its activities seem geared to couples or childless singles. Most importantly, don't be too proud to accept what help is offered.

If you are the spouse of the stay-at-home care-giver, you have a critical role in maintaining his or her sanity. Stay-at-home parents need to hear that they are important and desirable. They need adult conversation, not more prattle from the television. They need someone to take charge of the kids for a while, even when they're right there in the room. They need to go out for an evening with you, even to be taken away for a weekend if possible. They need to be sent cards and love notes for no particular reason. They need to be encouraged to develop their mind and skills; caring for the kids one night a week while they go to a class is considerate and would also give you an intense appreciation for the magnitude of their daily work.

Above all, those who raise children need to keep up their prayer life, because no one has all the answers, wisdom, and energy needed for the job—but God does. Don't forget: More than any other experience, this process will teach you about your relationship with God, who is the ultimate loving parent.

8. **Conflict on the home front: verbal (and other) warfare.** One of the most common and highly damaging contributors to chronic fatigue is a state of trench warfare at home. All too often those who have promised to "love, honor, and respect" at the altar find themselves in the midst of searing conflict before the honeymoon is over because they never learned how to address common (and inevitable) life issues while honoring and respecting their spouse's opinions and personhood. If the verbal battles continue unchecked, children soon learn to imitate this behavior, until the home becomes the most dangerous place in town. The ongoing prodding, accusing, put-downs, sarcasm, arguing, and in some cases physical fighting create an atmosphere that is draining and polluted. Since the patterns are usually ingrained and automatic, the combatants may be aware only of their constant dissatisfaction and fatigue.

Of all the contributors to chronic fatigue, this can be one of the toughest to resolve, because two or more people not only need to recognize the problem but also must learn to communicate without using verbal clubs. (However, one highly motivated person can model some constructive patterns for the others.) An astute counselor can facilitate this process, as can a mature couple or family whom you have observed relating in healthy ways. While it is not possible to detail all the principles involved in settling disagreements within the family in this book, the following basic concepts can serve as a foundation for those who desire to work on this important area.[5]

Mutual respect is an absolute necessity. Without respect on all sides, any relationship will ultimately deteriorate or become destructive. With mutual respect, it is possible to have an intense disagreement with another person without causing damage to the relationship or those who are affected by it. Respect acknowledges the ultimate worth of the other person—because he or she is made in God's image, not because of any other attributes or accomplishments—and affirms that worth in attitudes, words, and actions. If family members do not respect one another or if respect flows only in one direction, attempts to resolve issues are likely to be unsuccessful or hurtful. This fundamental problem must be addressed—usually in a counseling setting—if a marriage is going to survive and thrive through the years of raising children and beyond.

During a disagreement, conversation should focus on the issue and not the person. If Mom feels she needs more help with the kids in the evening, it isn't productive for her to begin the discussion with the statement "You care more about that TV than your own children!" If Dad is getting worried about the family budget, he won't get very far by saying, "All you ever do is spend the money I work so hard to bring home!" Once the issue is defined (How do we care for the kids when we're both tired? or How can we keep better track of our finances?), the focus can shift toward generating and evaluating a potential solution.

When an issue needs to be discussed, pick an appropriate time and place. The right time is not at the end of the day when energy is low and fuses may be short; not right before bed; not when anger is at a fever pitch; not when there isn't time to work through it; not when the TV is on, the phone is ringing, the kids are arguing, and the dog is barking. If it is clear that an issue needs to be addressed later, it's quite all right for either person to call time and say, "This isn't a good time to discuss this" or "I don't feel like talking about it right now"—as long as a specific time is set to talk about it in the very near future. The best time to talk is when both parties are rested, focused, and attentive. It's helpful to work through an issue in a place that is relatively free of distractions and interruptions. This may be a particular room, somewhere out in the yard, or a place away from home. Many couples do their best negotiating at a coffee shop or on a long walk.

Pray together before discussing the issue. Laying the issue before God can help keep it in perspective and reinforce your common ground. Be careful not to use this prayer time unfairly to express your viewpoint or claim God's backing for your side of the conflict. Prayer should be an exercise in humility, not a power play.

Each person must be able to express his or her viewpoint fully, without interruption. A key element of respect is listening carefully to what the other person is saying, without thinking about one's own response. One technique that encourages attentive listening involves picking an object (such as a pen) and stipulating that whoever holds it is entitled to speak without interruption. The other person

cannot say a word until the pen is passed, and the pen will not be passed until the person receiving it can summarize what was just said to the speaker's satisfaction—without argument, rebuttal, or editorial comment. If the listener doesn't get it right, the pen doesn't pass. This approach may seem awkward and ritualistic at first, but it is surprisingly effective at improving listening skills. Get in the habit of checking frequently to be sure that you understand what the other person is saying. "I hear you saying . . ."

Avoid "You . . ." statements—especially those containing the word *always, never, should,* or *shouldn't.* Replace them with statements that express your own feelings. "You *never* spend any time at home anymore!" essentially demands a rebuttal ("That's not true!"). In contrast, "It seems as if the kids and I are spending more evenings by ourselves than ever before, and it makes me feel lonely" is a straightforward observation and an expression of a genuine feeling. Similarly, a statement such as "You *shouldn't* make commitments for both of us without talking to me first!" is likely to provoke a defensive response. The one way in which a "you" statement can legitimately enter a conversation is in this form: "When you say (or do) _____, I feel _____ ." (For example, "When you make commitments for both of us without talking to me first, I feel as if my opinion doesn't count.") This type of statement can help one person understand how specific words or actions are affecting the other person.

Avoid "Why . . . ?" questions—especially those containing the word *always* or *never.* "Why do you always leave the back door open?" can be answered in only one of two ways: defensively ("I do not!") or sarcastically ("Because I'm an idiot!"). "Why . . . ?" questions automatically turn a discussion into a battle.

Avoid bringing up events from the distant past. Statements like "Here we go again!" or "This is just what you did on our vacation in 2002, when you . . ." are not helpful. If current problems are related to grievances from the past, then those specific concerns need to be discussed and resolved apart from any current problems.

Name-calling and other forms of insults are disrespectful and should be banned from all conversations within a family (or anywhere else). Verbal insults live in everyone's memory long after apologies have been made. One of the most powerful lessons that children can learn from their parents is how to disagree or be angry with a person without resorting to labeling, name-calling, or insults. Remember that body language (such as sighing and rolling the eyes), gestures, and tone of voice can communicate disrespect as powerfully as the most explicit insult.

When discussing an issue, participants should eventually explore possible courses of action. Questions like "What can I do to help you not feel so tired at the end of the day?" or "How can we make Sunday morning less hectic?" can lead to productive solutions. It may help to list a number of possibilities and then talk through the pros and cons of each one.

Realize that sometimes you may have to "agree to disagree," and that in doing so, neither person's viewpoint is to be subject to constant ridicule. This will mean compromising in some cases. There is usually, however, some solution that will allow for each person's needs to be met.

If your discussions of issues frequently deteriorate into shouting matches or glum stalemates, get some help. It takes courage and maturity to go to a counselor (or to a mature couple whom you know to be experienced in conflict resolution) to determine what goes wrong when disagreements arise in your home. Constructive suggestions from an unbiased third party, if acted upon consistently, can drastically improve the quality and outcome of these conversations.

9. **Unmet expectations and desires**. These can cause fatigue at any season of life, and they will never be detected during a medical examination. Generally, a person with unmet expectations thinks: *Things aren't turning out the way I had hoped.* Perhaps deep longings for companionship, children, recognition, or other measures of success have not been met, and there are no prospects on the horizon. Or the desires *have* been met, and they aren't all they were cracked up to be. The degree, the spouse, the home, the kids, the job, the raise, or the title isn't supplying

lasting contentment. The restless search for the next source of satisfaction continues—and fatigue may well accompany it.

This scenario is nothing new. Centuries ago King Solomon surveyed all that he had acquired: unimaginable wealth, political superiority, worthwhile building projects, education, and sexual satisfaction from one thousand partners. Yet he was still not at all satisfied:

> *I denied myself nothing my eyes desired;*
>
> *I refused my heart no pleasure.*
>
> *My heart took delight in all my work,*
>
> *and this was the reward for all my labor. . . .*
>
> *Yet when I surveyed all that my hands had done*
>
> *and what I had toiled to achieve,*
>
> *everything was meaningless, a chasing after the wind;*
>
> *nothing was gained under the sun. . . .*

> So I hated life, because the work that is done under the sun was grievous to me. All of it is meaningless, a chasing after the wind. . . . What does a man get for all the toil and anxious striving with which he labors under the sun? All his days his work is pain and grief; even at night his mind does not rest. This too is meaningless.
> (ECCLESIASTES 2:10-11, 17, 22-23)

This type of fatigue, this world-weariness, will not be resolved by medication, supplements, exercise, or other physical remedies. It is at its core spiritual and involves answering a primary question: Is true contentment generated internally, or is it the result of how things are going? What dictates mood—circumstances or a forward-looking, others-oriented, stable attitude sustained by God's transforming work at the core of our being?

The Scriptures use vivid imagery to portray the person who has a vibrant, energizing relationship with God:

> *He is like a tree planted by streams of water,*
>
> > *which yields its fruit in season*
> >
> > *and whose leaf does not wither.*
>
> *Whatever he does prospers.*
>
> (PSALM 1:3)

The image of the tree here is powerful, one worth comparing to our own day-to-day experience. It is solid, stable, and productive at the right time, constantly drawing life from the waters nearby. And we can be as secure as that tree as we develop our relationship with God and are transformed by Him.

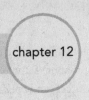

chapter 12

SOME FINAL THOUGHTS ON FATIGUE

Throughout this book, we describe symptoms and health hazards that arise from the frantic pace of our life. This point bears repeating as we conclude our look at fatigue. Jesus made a compelling offer: "Come to me, all you who are weary and burdened, and I will give you rest. Take my yoke upon you and learn from me, for I am gentle and humble in heart, and you will find rest for your souls. For my yoke is easy and my burden is light" (Matthew 11:28-30). Many who are "weary and burdened" are in fact straining and exhausted under yokes of their own making.

Far too many of us are overcommitted, underrested, and overstressed, and this often results in our feeling *tired*—physically, emotionally, and even spiritually. We fill our life with activities, most of which are good when considered individually. However, as they accumulate, they can lead to overload and then fatigue. Much of what we buy and accumulate is supposed to make our life simpler, easier, and less stressful. But in fact many of these items (including those that are supposed to save time or labor) actually consume more time, attention, resources, and energy than we ever intended.

We are the victims of hurry sickness as well, responding to an ongoing push to see and do more in less time. Like the drive to accumulate more possessions, some of this relentless pursuit is fueled by media and marketing. To own more and do more, we need to *make* more as well, so we push the throttle at work and often look for other sources of income while we're at it. Often the reward in the distance isn't financial but rather status and recognition, but these can capture our time and energy as effectively as any quest for a bigger paycheck. We seem unwilling to wait for anything anymore: Buy the big house *now*, get the new car *now*, take the exotic vacation *now*, and don't worry about that inevitable *pay later* part of the equation.

All the while, the most important things in life—relationships with God, family, and friends, not to mention time for exercise, sleep, reading, prayer, and other critical restoratives—are most often pushed to the background or out of the picture entirely. Our kids (who may have developed a frantic schedule of their own) not only suffer directly but may also see a mom and dad who can't say no. They may later mimic this example as adults.

In his books *Margin* and *The Overload Syndrome*, Dr.

Richard A. Swenson describes a process of "pruning the activity tree," which can be a major challenge for many families. But the reality is that we have limited resources of time, money, and energy, and we need to spend each of them wisely, with God as our adviser. We must realize that *no* can be a sacred word and have the courage to say it. We also need at times to ask ourselves why we feel compelled to have, to do, or to be something, to push ourselves and our families to the point of exhaustion.

We each have reserves to "run on empty" for a while, but we don't have an unlimited capacity to do so. To some degree this serves to remind us that we were designed to live within physical, mental, emotional, intellectual, and spiritual boundaries. We are not God, and one of the reminders of this reality is that we have limits. This may seem obvious, but too often our decisions reflect an unconscious assumption that *I can do it all!* Sooner or later, however, the challenges of life will bring us to the end of our intelligence, our knowledge, or our physical and emotional strength. Recognizing this may cause some to feel despair, but in fact this acknowledgment of our limits is the beginning of wisdom. Indeed, doing so *before* we reach the end of ourselves reflects even greater wisdom.

History, literature, and pop culture are abundant with would-be supermen and wonder women, but those who are not fictional or mythological inevitably prove to have feet of clay or chinks in their armor. Real people have been created for a relationship with God that is grounded on a humbling but also comforting reality: We are dependent on Him for every breath we take and every decision we make, and we need *each other* as well. The apostle Paul illustrates this mutual dependence with the analogy of a physical body whose various parts serve the whole:

Do not think of yourself more highly than you ought, but rather think of yourself with sober judgment, in accordance with the measure of faith God has given you. Just as each of us has one body with many members, and these members do not all have the same function, so in Christ we who are many form one body, and each member belongs to all the others.

(ROMANS 12:3-5)

God has arranged the parts in the body, every one of them, just as he wanted them to be. If they were all one part, where would the body be? As it is, there are many parts, but one body.

The eye cannot say to the hand, "I don't need you!" And the head cannot say to the feet, "I don't need you!" On the contrary, those parts of the body that seem to be weaker are indispensable, and the parts that we think are less honorable we treat with special honor. . . . God has combined the members of the body and has given greater honor to the parts that lacked it, so that there should be no division in the body, but that its parts should have equal concern for each other. If one part suffers, every part suffers with it; if one part is honored, every part rejoices with it.

(1 CORINTHIANS 12:18-26)

Our family, our friends, and our fellow believers in a community of faith fulfill different (and interdependent) roles in our life so that all can live more abundantly without feeling overburdened and worn out. Acknowledging our limits—the reality that we can't be and do everything—is not a liability or a sign of weakness. Instead, doing so provides opportunities to experience God's utter sufficiency and to serve one another in love—and in so doing, to avoid wearing ourselves out.

Endnotes

[1] K. Kroenke et al., "Chronic Fatigue in Primary Care: Prevalence, Patient Characteristics, and Outcome," *Journal of the American Medical Association* 260, no. 7 (August 19, 1988): 929–934. Abstract available at http://jama.ama-assn.org/cgi/content/abstract/260/7/929.

[2] Franklin Brown, Barlow Soper, and Walter C. Buboltz Jr., "Prevalence of Delayed Sleep Phase Syndrome in University Students," *College Student Journal* (September 2001). See http://www.findarticles.com/p/articles/mi_m0FCR/is_3_35/ai_80744660.

[3] Centers for Disease Control and Prevention, "Chronic Fatigue Syndrome." See http://www.cdc.gov/ncidod/diseases/cfs/about/what.htm.

[4] More information is available from the CFIDS Association of America (http://www.cfids.org), which both promotes research and disseminates educational material regarding this syndrome for patients, their families, and healthcare providers.

While most of the content of this organization's Web site is both informative and reasonable, note that some of its material and links dealing with alternative therapies steer patients toward approaches that are scientifically unsound or that have metaphysical underpinnings that neither Focus on the Family nor its Physicians Resource Council can endorse. It is important that individuals and families dealing with chronic fatigue syndrome discuss any treatment suggestions with their physician(s) and consider carefully the potential benefits and risks.

[5] The following suggestions have been adapted from the *Focus on the Family Complete Book of Baby and Child Care* (Wheaton, Ill.: Tyndale, 1997), 461–463.

Index

$6 REBATE

....

For a limited time you can get a $6.00 rebate on your purchase of *Complete Guide to Family Health, Nutrition, and Fitness*. Book must have been purchased in a retail store to qualify. Just return the completed rebate form, the original dated store receipt, and a photocopy of the UPC bar code from the book to: Complete Guide Rebate, Attn. Customer Service, 351 Executive Dr., Carol Stream, IL 60188.

Name: _____

Address: _____

_____

City:_____State:_____Zip:_____

Store where purchased: _____

E-mail address: _____

Signature: _____

GET THE *COMPLETE GUIDE TO FAMILY HEALTH, NUTRITION & FITNESS!*

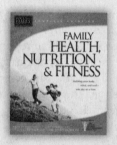

This comprehensive guide will help you take an active role in improving your health and well-being, as well as that of your entire family. It offers authoritative and current medical information in a convenient, easy-to-understand format. Taking a balanced, commonsense approach to the issue of health and wellness, this indispensable guide delivers helpful resources with an encouraging perspective.

OTHER FAITH AND FAMILY STRENGTHENERS FROM FOCUS ON THE FAMILY®

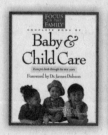

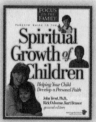

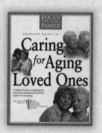